DR. CASS

The Lyme Disease Cure

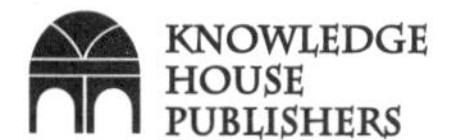

Second Edition
(Third Printing)

Printed in the United States of America

ISBN: 9781931078382

Disclaimer: This book is not intended as a substitute for medical diagnosis or treatment. Anyone who has a serious disease should consult a physician before initiating any change in treatment or before beginning any new treatment.

To order this or additional Knowledge House books call: 1-800-295-3737 or order via the web at: www.knowledgehousepublishers.com
Also see: www.cassingram.com

To get an order form send a SASE to:
Knowledge House Publishers

Printed in the United States of America

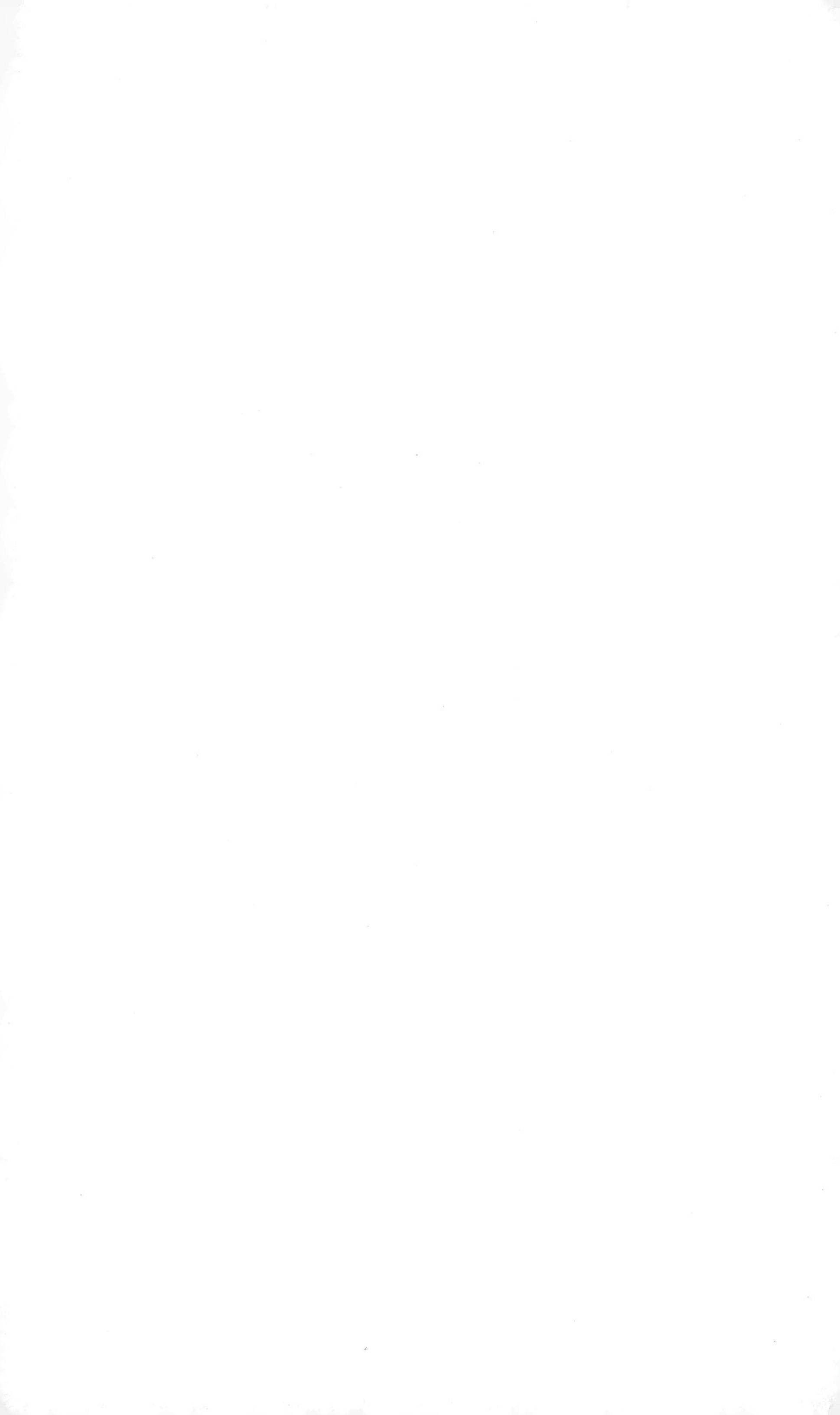

Table of Contents

	Foreward	7
	Introduction	11
Chapter One	**Nature as the Cure**	19
Chapter Two	**Internal Attack**	29
Chapter Three	**Biogerms on the Loose**	37
Chapter Four	**Conspiracy to Kill**	45
Chapter Five	**Lab Freaks and Bizarre Yeasts**	57
Chapter Six	**Danger in the Woods**	67
Chapter Seven	**Preventive Medicine**	90
Chapter Eight	**Is Lyme Weaponized Syphilis?**	99
Chapter Nine	**Neurological Lyme**	111
Chapter Ten	**Natural Cures to the Rescue**	133
Chapter Eleven	**Complications and Syndromes**	151
Chapter Twelve	**Co-Infections**	167
Chapter Thirteen	**Do's and Don'ts in Fighting Lyme**	177
Chapter Fourteen	**Nutrients Against Lyme**	193
Chapter Fifteen	**Recipes and Menus**	203
Chapter Sixteen	**The Lyme Child**	243
Chapter Seventeen	**Conclusion**	249
	Appendix A	257
	Bibliography	265
	Index	268

Foreward

No doubt, it is far easier to speak of any issue not from mere book knowledge but, rather, from personal experience. This is surely the case in regard to medical diseases, for doctors as well as patients. Nowhere could this be more true than with Lyme disease. It has been denied for years that it is such a potentially ominous issue—a true global pandemic. Since this disease has become manifested the medical profession has been less than forthcoming, surely less than honest regarding it. As a result, Lyme has not been taken as seriously as it should be.

People have let their guard down, especially in the medical profession, the warnings of caution are not sufficient. Prevention should be a national issue. Yet, it is not. Instead there's infighting about what kind of therapy to give and how long to give it. As a result, there is no cooperation, no global awareness campaign. Thus, people have contracted the disease when it could have been prevented. Plus, there is no open-mindedness to any degree, so that all potential modalities of treatment are offered to patients.

After suffering a number of tick bites I had become a sort of expert on just what could be contracted directly from ticks. Usually, though, these were diseases other than Lyme or, perhaps, a less severe form than the modern type. Even so, once I did develop single joint disease plus cardiac symptoms, the latter representing a possible case of cardiac Lyme. Yet, it was rapidly resolved through relatively aggressive use of natural spice-based germicides, edible oil of wild oregano in a super-strength form, along with an aromatic water known as wild juice of oregano. It didn't take long for the symptoms to be purged, about two weeks, and the more aggressive I was in the use of such natural cures the more rapidly the syndrome responded. This was some 10 years before I had written this book. There were no sequelae of any kind.

Yet, even with contracting multiple tick bites over the years, I had never endured anything that was absolutely dire, in fact, so much so that little could be done to reverse it, at least not until now. This time it was different. I suffered the bite of all bites, in this case by a stealth pathogen from the unseen, the miniscule nymphal form of the so-called deer tick, *Ioxides scapularis*.

What a cataclysm it was, one that, seemingly, even I with all I knew could not readily stop. It was as if all the most devastating and deadly aspects of such a disaster worked in sync. The fact that a tick bite occurred was not realized, at least not until the infection was well established. Why? It was because of the location of the bite, not on any visible part of the body but, rather, in the middle of the back. Unknowingly, I had been sleeping on that engorged tick, night after night. Nor could I have known that in those oppressive days of the disease's origin what was systematically developing on my back. This was a massive bullseye rash. I simply had no idea, not until I felt like I was dying, as if burning up alive, as if losing my mind.

The most intensive burning was on the skin. "What is this horrible sensation on my back?," I thought. "It's burning so badly. What is it?" After turning around and looking in the mirror, there it was, a bullseye rash the size of a flattened football.

It was now too late *not* to suffer. While the tick was long gone, who knows how long it was there? Who knows what it injected? Whatever that injection was it had already attacked my brain and spinal cord. The suffering was nothing less than horrific, so agonizing and extreme that it is hard to describe. It was also terrifying. Yes, terrifying, even for such an experienced man of the wilderness.

During the most difficult phases of this cataclysm many thoughts went through my mind, especially when the illness proved so resistant to the therapeutic approach that was applied. It was obvious that the pathogen(s) was attacking the most critical organ systems of the body, particularly the bloodstream, immune organs, and central nervous system. "Would it be possible to even survive this?," I wondered. "Couldn't this have been prevented? It would have been so much easier not to go through this pain, this agony." Yet, it was not to be so. It had to be this way. *It was meant to be.* Otherwise, I would never have known, never been able to pen these words, never been capable of probing and discovering the deeper truths. Then and only then could the ultimate result be achieved. This is to share—and to care—as well as to shed light on all that could be shed, including the necessary love: for all those who have likewise suffered.

In fact, there was no other way to consider it. There had to be a reason to suffer this immensely. It must be for the greater good, for the higher road. It must be to do what can be done to aid humankind—what could be greater than that?

Humankind: what kind of word is this? *Human-kind*. Kindness to the fellow human? The milk of *human kind-ness* to those desperately in need? To those who are suffering in a way that is so dire that it cannot even be described, who are in need of help with no hope in sight and no idea where to turn? Surely, this is the higher purpose, perhaps, the only one, for human existence.

It is a high road: to share love and kindness to others and to do so without any need for return or reward. There could be no better realm nor any superior reward. To this end this book is dedicated, to all those have suffered endlessly and who wish to suffer no more.

Introduction

There is a vast epidemic which is afflicting millions of Americans as well as other uncountable people globally. Epidemic is not the right word. Instead, it is a pandemic. Moreover, unlike the typical pandemic, which is transitory, this is continuous. This is Lyme disease, one of the most dreaded and destructive diseases known.

No one can fully fathom the scope of this illness. In many respects as a disease it is unprecedented. Here is a condition which virtually out of nowhere has fully established itself, disrupting and even destroying the lives of millions of people yearly, many of whom were previously in excellent health.

Continuous pandemic means that, internationally, the infectious process remains active. In other words, it doesn't wax and wane, as do flu pandemics. This is demonstrated by the statistics in the United States and Europe alone. In the USA there are an estimated 300,000 new cases each year. Imagine it: 300,000. What a monstrous number it is. This means that in over a decade there will be some three million cases, in two decades, six million, and in over a thirty year period an incredible 12 million new cases. That amounts to nearly 4% of the total population of this country.

The 300,000 cases represent Lyme spirochete infections only. In the United States there are dozens of other infectious syndromes caused by ticks. Reasonably stated, in the USA alone there are likely a half million new cases of diseases due to tick germ infestation annually. In this country there is no other epidemic of such a magnitude known.

It ultimately represents the unfathomable: a half million cases yearly of people who are sickened by not merely the typical pathological agents, such as hospital acquired germs, colds, and the flu, but, rather, the atypical if not aberrant. These are the pathogens of vermin, that is germs that exist in mice, shrews, rats, ground squirrels, and other species of the rodent family. Such animals are far more likely the original source of tick-borne germs than larger mammals such as deer, elk, cattle, racoons, skunks, and opossums.

Ticks are merely the vectors, with the white-tailed deer acting as the intermediate host. Humans are the end-stage host. Actually, they are the ultimate victims as they rarely transmit the disease. Furthermore, they have little to no capacity to resist the onset of the infection.

In Europe it is no better. Lyme and various other tick-source germ infections infest both the United Kingdom and countries on the continent.

Make no mistake about it this is a horror upon humanity of the most extreme degree. How truly aggressive the Lyme pathogen is, capable of destroying the health of perfectly normal people. Virtually no disease could be as fearsome as this, so incapacitating, so destructive that it wipes out lives, literally.

Almost everyone seemingly knows about this condition, especially people in the United States. Along with Europe this is where the majority of cases occur. Americans have heard numerous stories of the devastation caused by Lyme and how it ruins people's health and lives. They may know of an individual personally who has been afflicted. Or, they may be victims themselves.

Regardless, for a chronic disease it is also in a league of its own. The condition can drain a person of his/her entire capacity, all one's strength being exhausted and dissipated. Because of the joint attack it can incapacitate the individual and/or make such a one's life miserable. The disease involves an attack on virtually every region of the body, although the joints, heart, and nervous system suffer the brunt of the damage.

Now, ominously, in North America, as well as Europe, this tick-borne disease represents the most commonly occurring of all insect-induced, that is vector-induced, diseases known. While it is now established that the disease is transmitted through a number of means the so called black-legged deer tick, known medically as *Ixodes scapularis*, is by far the most common perpetrator.

In certain states of the United States it is such a horror that it is beyond a pandemic. Examples include Connecticut, Pennsylvania, and Massachusetts. Connecticut is a prime example of the extreme nature of the infestation. As the state of origin, it appears to have the disease in the highest known incidence and greater pathology than anywhere else in the world. Says T. Moorcroft, D.O., who practices in Berlin, CT, there are reportedly some 122 cases of Lyme which develop yearly per 100,000 people. Yet, as he makes clear this is not a truly accurate representation. According to the CDC a mere 10% of actual cases of Lyme are known. In other words, for every case that is known there are nine others who have the disease but are unaware of it, whether symptomatic or not. Nor do their doctors know they have it. That means that, for instance, in Connecticut for every 100,000 people there are 1,000 new cases which develop annally, making this, perhaps, the greatest pandemic of all time. That's at least one percent of all people in the state, which is huge. The same holds true nationwide. There are between 20,000 to 30,000 reported cases of the disease yearly, and, by the way, that's just Lyme, not the co-infections. That means that, as stated previously, yearly, there are up to 300,000 new cases which is massive, actually, monstrous beyond belief. That dwarfs all other epidemics into absolute insignificance.

What could cause such devastation? It is a tick which is barely visible to the naked eye. This tick injects into the human body unusually destructive types of bacteria known as spirochetes. Even so, it should be re-named the "rodent tick," as the causative germs thrive primarily in this population of mammals, not deer.

The spirochete which causes Lyme is known medically as *Borrelia burgdorferi.* The term borrelia is descriptive. It indicates the capacity to "bore." This spirochete is a cork screw-appearing organism. The fact is the cork-screw structure is responsible for much of its destructive powers. It gives it the capacity to vigorously invade the tissues like no other germ. It's mechanism of action is based on a novel structure. On one end of the bacterium there is an anatomical mechanism for latching on to the involved tissue. The latching is necessary to give it leverage. Then, through its spike-like head it bores its way into the tissues, just like a screw being screwed forcibly into a wall.

Too, the term Lyme is descriptive. It denotes the regions of the original outbreak. These regions are Lyme and Old Lyme, Connecticut.

The name 'burgdorferi' is also readily explained. It is merely the last name of the man who discovered the causative agent, Willy Burgdorferi, who in 1981 isolated it from a deer tick. That research was an outcome of the novel origin of this new epidemic, where investigators sought to find the source of the pathogen causing spotty outbreaks of infectious arthritis in humans.

Because of their highly invasive capacities cork-screw organisms are capable of causing vast damage. The attack of the Lyme bacillus on the joints is particularly dire, although why it specifically attacks these body components is largely unexplained. However, it is now believed that the spirochete feeds preferentially on connective tissue, the main structural component found in joints. It actually invades the deepest recesses of the joint. Thereafter, it seems to selectively hide in the joint capsule, where it causes significant inflammation as well as tissue destruction. Also, through a mechanism yet to be determined it causes rheumatoid arthritis-like damage, actual joint destruction. Moreover, Lyme arthritis is nearly as stubborn as the standard type of rheumatoid arthritis, being resistant to the majority of medical treatments. In Lyme, though, the degree of deformity is less severe than that occurring in rheumatoid arthritis.

Yet, this attack by the Lyme spirochete is only a part of the debacle. There are a wide range of other germs which may also infect the tick bite victim, including other spirochetes yet to be described and also a wide range of other bacteria. Additionally, ticks may inject a variety of pathogenic parasites and viruses. Germ-induced conditions associated with Lyme are known as co-infections. Those co-infections caused by parasites, notably protozoans, are particularly disconcerting and relatively common, as are infestations by another key category of bacteria known as rickettsia.

Now, regarding the viruses injected by ticks these are also of great concern. A number of these cause encephalitis syndromes. These newly discovered co-infections will also be covered in this book.

There is another infectious agent which may infect tick bite victims which is neither a bacteria nor a virus. This is mycoplasma, particularly the species, *Mycoplasma fermentans*. Still other agents of infestation include the bacterium ehrlichia and also bartonella.

As for overall pathology, though, Lyme takes precedence. This may largely be the result of the germ's highly unusually potent invasive powers. It may also be a consequence of yet another propensity, which is its ability to evade the immune system. This germ operates by stealth. Plus, as a result of its deep, burrowing action into tissues, especially the bones, brain, and spinal cord, it is difficult to eradicate. Moreover, because of such burrowing inflammation results, which adds an additional burden upon the process of achieving a cure.

Too, because of the nature of its infective powers despite an ongoing immune response against the pathogen it can persist, often for long periods. Without proper treatment this persistence could be for a lifetime. This is partly the result of another aspect of borrelia, which is its capacity to morph into a different form: a kind of dormant element. This dormant element is also difficult for the immune system to recognize and thus eradicate. It is an encysted form of the Lyme bacillus, which antibiotics, for instance, cannot kill. Therefore, even with seemingly successful orthodox therapy the Lyme may resurge upon the release of the germ from its encysted form. Such a release may often result from stress or poor diet or, possibly, the contraction of an infection, like the flu.

It does seem almost beyond belief and hopeless. In this regard what is the victim to do? Such a one typically can only rely on the standard treatment offered by orthodox medicine. Even so, with orthodox medical treatment what can be done to prevent and treat Lyme resurgence? Additionally, what can be done in cases where an individual is sensitive to antibiotics or where the antibiotic therapy fails to achieve eradication? Moreover, again, what about that encysted form? How dire; what can the tick bite victim do to purge that from the body?

Fortunately, there is hope. That hope comes from wild nature. The godly medicines *can* cure this disease. Incredibly, there are a wide range of natural complexes which are capable of obliterating such germs. There are also certain natural cures capable of destroying both forms, the active and encysted types. The most potent of these are natural medicines that few people would even realize. These are medicines which are aggressive germicides. A germicide is capable of killing a wide range of germs, in some cases virtually all known germs. These natural germicides are the wild spice oils, particularly oil of wild oregano.

Chapter One

Nature is the Cure

Does nature provide the cure for Lyme? Or, are synthetic drugs the answer? Or, are antibiotic agents the sole means of hope? A cursory review of the literature demonstrates that by no means are drugs an efficient or even reliable cure.

Consider what was discovered by medical researchers as early as the late 1980s. In *Arthritis and Rheumatism*, 1987, a number of clinical cases were described, which demonstrate this point. According to the investigators R.J. Dattwyler and J.J. Halperin some five cases were evaluated for their response to the then standard treatment, tetracycline-class antibiotics. The patients, it was demonstrated, had despite receiving tetracycline therapy early in the illness "developed significant late complications." These after-treatment manifestations included paralysis of the facial nerve, damage to the nerves to the feet and arms (peripheral neuropathy), chronic fatigue, and alteration in mental state. Incredibly, the researchers concluded even in this early date that by no means is the orthodox therapy effective and that, rather, it was so ineffective that it should be "reconsidered" as a dependable treatment for early Lyme.

Antibiotics have their place, yet clearly it takes much more than mere drugs to resolve the majority of cases of spirochete infestation. Make no mistake about it this is a difficult microbe to eradicate, even with the most potent medications. So, it is reasonable to pursue the benefits of all modalities of therapy, including the full spectrum of natural remedies—wild nature to the rescue. Even so, time is of essence in order to properly treat spirochete infestation. The longer the agent has an opportunity to infect the body, unopposed, the more devastating are the consequences. Extracts of wild oregano and other spices are the answer for Lyme disease. Really, mere spices? For instance, oregano is a pizza spice, right? How could it also be a potent medicine capable of curing infectious diseases such as Lyme?

In fact, the pizza spice cannot achieve such results. Often, this spice is derived from non-oregano species such as Mexican sage, known botanically as *Lippia gravolens*. This can be seen by reading the oregano spice labels; it often says Mexican oregano. Too, it may be Spanish or Moroccan in source, a species known as *Thymus capitatus*. True wild oregano is actual Origanum species of a wide range, including the Greek type *Origanum heraculoticum* and various others. These medicinal types of oregano plants grow wild in the high Mediterranean mountains up to 12,000 feet above sea level.

Despite that high, seemingly infertile area it thrives in such an environment, growing poorly if at all in lower elevations. On dirt it fails to thrive. In fact, when forced to grow on farm land, the plant becomes diseased and even becomes contaminated with mold. Thus, avoid all sources of oil of wild oregano derived from farm-raised plants.

Truly wild oregano grows, impressively, above the tree line, nourishing itself on white, calcareous rock. Without the white rock environment this type of wild oregano is incapable of growing.

Additionally, commercial oregano is often adulterated and is mixed with weeds as well as dried leaves of trees. This dilutes its medicinal powers. Another reason that this is not medicinal is the fact that it is irradiated, apparently, routinely so by FDA policy. In health food stores there is, though, non-irradiated oregano, and this is a superior choice over the commercial type. Yet, it is not sufficiently potent to reverse diseases of the scope of Lyme. For this far more potent types of wild oregano must be used.

The key material to utilize in the reversal of Lyme disease is the wild oregano oil. This is an extract made from the true wild oregano species that grow on the mountain tops in the Mediterranean. Oil of wild oregano is the steam extract of this remote source wild oregano.

Only mountain-grown wild oregano and/or its extracts should be procured as a means of natural support in Lyme disease. It is this type of wild oregano which is entirely safe to use in tick-induced infections and which can, therefore, be used daily as well as in unlimited quantities.

Be sure to purchase only such an extract from the remote source, wild mountain oregano species. Too, it must be derived from the real, true oregano, the same type that is used in Mediterranean cooking. Avoid cheap imitations made from false oregano, including those made from Mexican sage and *Thymus capitatus* as well as those listed as *Origanum vulgare*. Too, for the protocols in this book avoid the consumption of oregano oil produced from farm-raised sources as well as genetically engineered spice.

Incredible as it may seem there actually is genetically engineered oregano and, therefore, oregano oil on the market. Such corruption is known as GMOs, which stands for "genetically modified organisms." This means that this type of oregano, like the food of the same category, is tainted with foreign genes. In this case the oregano is injected with bacterial material from the germ *Pseudomonas auregenosa*. The purpose of such an injection is to provoke the plant to increase its levels of a key active ingredient, known as carvacrol.

All such oregano plants are raised in an environment that is unnatural to the plant, that is on standard soils at low elevations. In order to maintain the growth of such aberrant plants, often, herbicides and pesticides are used. Therefore, all oregano oil derived from GMO-tainted plants is inherently corrupt.

Typically, such GMO-based oregano oils have carvacrol levels of 80% or higher. In contrast, natural-source oregano has a carvacrol level of between 55% and 75%. Only small amounts in nature bear levels of 80% or higher. That level of the active ingredient in nature is actually quite rare.

Yet, carvacrol is only one of a number of active ingredients. In the true wild oregano oil from edible spice the number of such active ingredients often exceeds 30. In contrast, the number of such ingredients in genetically engineered versions is as low as 12. Independent testing of brands off health food store shelves conducted by a nutritional supplement company (North American Herb & Spice, the original maker of edible oil of wild oregano), proves a dire issue. In Canada and the United States some 35% of all brands tested are derived from genetically altered (GMO) oregano. Such brands have high carvacrol levels, while bearing a reduced number of other key active ingredients, that is those miscellaneous synergistic compounds naturally occurring in the oil, less than half that seen in true wild oregano oil.

This means that there are a number of commonly available oregano oil supplements on the market that are corrupted with GMOs, in other words, bacterial genes and proteins. In nature oregano or its extracted oil is never contaminated with such aberrant genes.

One key means of determining quality is price. High-grade oil of wild oregano derived from 100% handpicked, wild spice is often twice the price of imitation brands.

As it can be readily imagined wild oil of oregano is surely a potent substance. It takes 100 pounds of the wild oregano dried spice to produce a pound of oil. That's about 500 pounds of the fresh, undried spice. Some 500 pounds to get 5 pounds: how absolutely potent and vigorous it is. In a pure, undiluted form it is too potent for human consumption. The original research on animals and humans regarding its germicidal properties was done with an emulsified form, that is oil of wild oregano in a base of extra virgin olive oil. The extra virgin olive oil emulsion in the animal studies was far more well tolerated than the undiluted oil, which was far too aggressive, causing significant gastric and intestinal irritation, leading in test mice even to fatality. Based on that research, largely conducted at Georgetown University, only such an emulsion can be recommended for daily or regular consumption.

How it works

This natural spice extract operates via a number of mechanisms. One of its key mechanisms is dissolution. In other words, it is capable of dissolving germs. This is true of both the active and encysted forms. This is why no germ can resist its action. A germ is mostly water. If the outer coating of such an organism is dissoluted, then, its water content is spilled out. Under such circumstances there is no way the germ can survive. Thus, through regular use of spice oils the pathogens which cause Lyme can be thoroughly purged. Another mechanism is direct damage to the intracellular components. Essentially, the spice oils disable the internal workings of the germs, resulting in their destruction.

Other natural medicines to the rescue

Oil of wild oregano can be safely used in concert with orthodox medical treatment, including antibiotics.The same is true of other spice oil-based germicides. All such spice oils have broad, destructive effects against a wide range of germs, including the Lyme bacillus. The main natural food-based spice oil supplements, which are ideal in the treatment of Lyme and various co-infections, are the wild oil of oregano, the multiple spice dessicated spice oil concentrate made from oils of wild oregano, wild sage, cinnamon oil, and cumin oil as well as wild juice of oregano. The wild juice of oregano is the steam-extracted oregano hydrosol. Additionally, it may be of value to consume the whole crude herb combined with its associated edible wild herbal berry, *Rhus coriaria*. Such supplements offer real hope for Lyme victims, who are under siege and who have few options from which to choose.

For the inflammation associated with Lyme another key spice oil complex is wild turmeric extract. Such turmeric extract is superior to the commercial types. Other turmeric supplements are derived from the farm-raised spice. When raised in this manner, often, a considerable amount of pesticides and herbicides are used. Residues of these noxious chemicals may be found in turmeric, since the spice readily absorbs fat soluble compounds.

Yet, another issue relates to processing. Virtually all commercially available turmeric supplements, whether found in the mass market or health food stores, are solvent extracted. The main solvent used for such extraction is hexane, a gasoline-like substance. This is never the case with wild turmeric extract, available as sublingual drops and gelcaps. It is extracted using only steam and carbon dioxide. Regarding the latter this is known as supercritical extraction.

Once again, since they are foods the true wild oregano-based supplements, along with other complexes derived from spices, are safe for human consumption. They can be used as the focus of treatment. Yet, impressively, they can also be used along with any medical treatment *if a person so chooses.*

Even so, through the use of any potent germ-killing substance there is a key issue, which must be addressed. This relates to the potential killing power of not only the harmful bacteria but also the good ones, the latter being known as probiotics. Since these compounds kill bacteria, there is a risk that they will kill not only the unhealthy ones but also the good ones: the probiotics. This is a definite issue, especially when antibiotics and antiseptics, that is germicides, are taken in unison. In this regard it is essential to combat the killing effect with probiotics. This is in the form of supplements but also probiotic-rich foods.

Yet, in modest doses wild oil of oregano is non-toxic to the good bacteria. In one study it was determined that small doses, like a few drops daily or a few capsules of the whole, crude herb actually enhanced the growth of probiotics. However, in large doses their growth was temporarily suppressed, although upon discontinuing the oregano oil those bacteria eventually regenerated. In the types of doses needed to clear tick-injected germs from the body it is likely that the good bacteria will be, to a degree, killed. Thus, any such supplementation should be combined with the intake of probiotics.

There are dozens of probiotic brands/supplements available on the market. One particularly ideal formula is based upon extensive research conducted in the European Union. Known as Ecologic 500, this formula consists of a combination of nine different bacteria, including novel forms such as *Bifidobacterium infintis*, lactis, and longum, along with *Lactobacillus acidophilus*, and plantarum, among others. The great value of this formula for human health has been demonstrated through a number of scientific studies. These studies have shown that Ecologic 500 has an unusually potent capacity to achieve the ultimate result desired for such bacteria, which is implantation. With other formulas, it was determined, the bacteria simply colonized in the intestine but were gradually lost out of the body.

There is another novel feature of this formula, which is the source. The bacteria in this formulation are derived not from animal or human gut, as are other supplements, but, rather, plants. That's right, this bacterial blend is derived from the ultimate source of healthy bacteria such as grasses; it is these sources which are the safest for human consumption as well as the most potent in terms of achieving vigorous implantation.

As additional sources of probiotics fermented foods also are invaluable for combating this killing effect. In regard to antibiotic treatment some doctors recommend such foods alone as the means of neutralizing any die-off of the good bacteria. The best food sources of healthy bacteria include natural wholefood yogurt—that is yogurt made from unprocessed, whole milk—sauerkraut, quark, and kefir. Ideally, regarding yogurt, it should come from organic sources.

In particular, if they achieve implantation, probiotics do cause an improvement in health. They surely cause a balancing in digestion and elimination. Plus, their regular intake has a bolstering effect on the immune system as well as liver function. These bacteria are highly industrious, producing their own versions of antibiotics, one of which is known, appropriately, as acidophilin. They also produce a wide range of vitamins, including the B complex and vitamin K.

Efficiency of cure: antibiotics or natural, wild extracts?

Moreover, in most cases of Lyme it is essential to utilize such a natural, therapeutic approach, which is made clear by the nature of Lyme and various tick-source co-infections. Furthermore, in Lyme and Lyme-like syndromes in most instances the body is dealing with a multitude of infections, that is a number of organisms which are simultaneously infecting the body. How can antibiotics, which are aimed at single organisms, be the most efficient cure in such circumstances? In fact, in the case of tick bite diseases they cannot be the ultimate treatment offering such efficiency. For instance, the main class of drugs used in Lyme disease, the tetracycline antibiotics, do not kill a number of the co-infecting agents, for example, babesia. Nor can such drugs kill the wide range of viruses which may be injected by these insects. Nor are they capable of killing molds and fungi. In contrast, antiseptics—or germicides, such as oil of wild oregano and other spice oil complexes—obliterate the entire range of tick-induced pathogens, including viruses, molds, fungi, bacteria, and protozoans.

In contrast to antibiotics wild spice oil-based germicides don't discriminate between even the various types of bacteria themselves, that is they are not specialist drugs. Rather, they destroy the full range of such germs, all the different species of spirochetes, rickettsia, and more. For instance, in one study conducted by the Pasteur Institute oregano oil was found to do the untenable. It actually sterilized septic, that is sewage, water. The investigation, conducted in 1918 by Cavel and colleagues, determined that after adding the oil to the water in a one to 1000 dilution the septic water was so thoroughly neutralized that it was impossible to reculture any germs. Clearly, oil of wild oregano is a germicide, not an antibiotic. This makes it ideal in the treatment of Lyme, in fact, from a natural point of view the treatment of choice.

It is, after all, all about choice. This is especially the case with diseases which are chronic in nature and which medicine has no means of absolutely curing. Such is the case with countless tick bite victims who, despite orthodox treatment, remain burdened with their symptoms and diseases. In such cases the use of the protocols in this book will prove ideal and in many instances lifesaving.

Nevertheless, one of the keys to reversing Lyme is the intake of wild foods—and wild-source supplements. This is based upon one of the premises of this book, which is the fact that wild animals despite infestation with tick-borne germs are relatively immune to the syndromes developed by humans. The spice oil complexes and their extracted oils are largely wild. So are the probiotic bacteria derived from wild plants. As a source for wild foods and wild-source supplements, see www.americanwildfoods.com

Chapter Two

Internal Attack

Like other systemic diseases, such as arthritis, lupus, and diabetes, Lyme represents a widespread attack on the entire body. The same, though, is true of all other tick-based infestations, including the various co-infections associated with the Lyme tick bite. As stated by T. M. Grier in his book *Lyme Disease Survival Manual* the disease constitutes a condition which is "multi-system," meaning it can affect virtually every tissue and organ of the body. In some cases, Grier makes clear, it causes a mild disorder while in others it can prove crippling, even deadly. It is simply the nature of the infectious agent, the spirochete, which upon entering the body readily populates and then "spreads," initially to mainly the joints and nervous system.

One of the direst aspects of the disease, he notes, relates to the capacity, or lack of such a capacity, to readily diagnose it. In fact, doctors routinely miss it despite suspect symptoms. Additionally, there is no absolute blood test for Lyme. It is possible to test negative yet still have it. It is also possible to test positive and have no symptoms.

The criteria for the diagnosis of Lyme is often made using the CDC's surveillance case definition for the disease. This includes a testing procedure based on both an antibody screening and the Western blot test, the latter serving as confirmation. Even so, these tests miss up to 50% of patients who have active infection.

One of the biggest dilemmas with Lyme disease testing is that the best tests available are blood tests, while the Lyme disease-causing agents do not live in the blood. A recently published study of monkeys experimentally infected with *Borrelia burgdorferi* found that the C_6 antibody test gave false negative results in *all* the monkeys treated with antibiotics, along with over half those that were untreated. Currently, there are no blood tests that will determine with certainty the existence or lack of existence of Lyme spirochete infestation. Signs and symptoms, along with a history of exposure, are, thus, more reliable as evidence than blood tests. In this regard it is important to emphasize that a negative blood test may not mean anything. A person could still have active Lyme disease; it may mean merely that the subject's immune system is not producing antibodies to borrelia.

Further complicating the issue is the fact that in some cases the symptoms occur within days of the actual bite, while in others these symptoms may not occur until years later. Therefore, countless thousands of people suffer with the disease with its wide-ranging and often destructive symptoms and have no idea that it is Lyme, which is the cause.

Consider the circumstances. A tick bites a human and injects is fluids/secretions, including gut fluids and saliva. The spirochete then enters the blood stream and lymphatic system, where it overpopulates. It then infects critical organ systems. As a result, the bite victim develops a devastating illness. Even so, it may not be Lyme that is the key element. Rather, it could have been any of a wide range of other pathogenic agents that created the sickness, including mycoplasma, bartonella, ehrlichia, and parasites. There are potentially hundreds of destructive pathogens in the blood, gut fluids, and saliva of ticks. Consider what they feed upon, the lowest animals of the low: rodents, among others. Thus, the essential element is, "Could there have been a tick bite that led to the person's condition, any tick bite, anywhere in the world?"

Additionally, it should be asked, "Did the condition originate in the spring or summer or, perhaps, early fall? Was joint pain or swelling—or immobility—an early or presenting manifestation of the syndrome?" Too, "Was fatigue or absolute exhaustion associated?" and, importantly, "Was there a migrating rash or any kind of unusual rash associated with the illness?" Another key to making the diagnosis is as follows: "Was swelling, pain, and/or immobility in a single joint, like a knee, ankle, or elbow, the main presenting symptom?" The sudden onset of such symptoms in late spring and early summer, as well as mid- and/or late summer, is highly indicative of the development of Lyme.

Regarding the joints the signs and symptoms of bacterial infection are well established. Astute internists and family practitioners know that if a person presents with joint pain, inflammation, and swelling in a single joint, it is bacterial arthritis until proven otherwise. Of course, the exception is the person who has sustained direct injury to such a joint, for instance, a sports-related trauma or a fall.

Too, as a general rule the single joint presentation is typical of spirochete-induced disease. For instance, syphilis may initially present as single joint damage and inflammation. The single joint presentation, though, may suddenly change, transforming into multiple joint involvement. The spirochete may migrate from one major joint to the other. It is likely that this migration is mediated through the nervous system. In this regard the germ may migrate through the nerve sheath via axoplasmic flow. Upon reaching the joint it launches its invasive attack. It, without doubt, lives and thrives in the central nervous system.

Once again, how does it present? It may begin in the knee and end up for no explanation elsewhere, like the elbow, hip, or ankle. Less commonly, there may even be migration to the TMJ (temporomandibular joint) or neck. The spirochete attack upon the TMJ region can be extreme, leading to the inability to properly open the mouth and/or chew. Moreover, the Lyme bacillus is one of the few germs which can cause such a presentation. It is truly bizarre and, furthermore, defies explanation.

Yet, the question is in the event of a tick bite is the Lyme spirochete the culprit for such presentations, or is it some other tick-borne germ? Often, this question may prove impossible to define. To a degree it is irrelevant, at least in terms of the premises described here. The natural treatment for all tick-related diseases is essentially the same, that is regardless of the infectious agent(s) involved.

There is yet another way tick bites can manifest, though it is far from exclusive of Lyme. This is tick-induced paralysis. The paralysis can be the primary initial presentation, one that is even more dire than joint inflammation. It comes on suddenly, often associated with a headache. The headache is a sign of infestation by the tick-injected germs into the brain and, consequently, spinal cord. It represents a kind of tick-induced encephalitis and may be associated with a stiff neck. Suddenly, the leg and/or arm go numb, and the person cannot move them. The face can also go numb as the initial presenting symptom combined with facial muscle paralysis. Such presentations are typical of bites not only by the black-legged Lyme tick but also the red-bodied wood tick.

The paralysis is usually unilateral. Yet, in some extreme cases it may be full-body, that is paralysis of the body below the waist involving both legs. It is a Guillain-Barré-like presentation. In fact, the tick-induced paralysis is often misdiagnosed as this condition or, perhaps, multiple sclerosis. It may also be misdiagnosed as ALS (Lou Gehrig's disease). Any such paralysis is a likely consequence of tick bites along the occipital region, the neck, and the scalp.

Yet another presentation is paralysis of the muscles of the face, known as Bell's palsy. This palsy is a sign that the spirochete has infected the sheath of the fifth cranial nerve. This may be the only presenting symptom of a tick bite. It is a common presenting symptom of both deer tick and wood tick bites. In the sudden onset of Bell's palsy, that is facial palsy of the muscles of one side of the face, occurring in the summer tick-induced disease must be suspected. Such paralysis is a sign that the tick-injected germs have infested the central nervous system—the spinal cord, its fluids, the brain, its fluids, and the nerves arising from these organs. In virtually all such cases spirochete infestation is likely, not just in Lyme disease but also potentially multiple others. This explains the paralysis-induced by the bite of non-Lyme wood ticks such as those which are commonly found in the woods of middle America and Canada.

Modern research has proven that, untreated, such tick-induced conditions lead to widespread damage of the nervous system. The tick-spread germs, notably the Lyme spirochete, as well as the spirochetes found in the bellies of wood ticks, attack the nerve cells, causing them to die. If sufficient numbers of such cells are killed, then, paralysis results.

Then, too, the medical treatment for such paralysis is problematic. Often, highly potent drugs, steroids and the like, are prescribed. These drugs merely suppress the function of the immune system, as well as the function and operations of the nervous system. The symptoms may thus improve, yet this is not the case with the infection. This immune suppression merely drives the germs deeper into the tissues, where they remain to launch their next assault at any opportune moment. Therefore, despite any temporary benefits, potent immunosuppressive drugs, such as steroids and methotrexate, should not be taken for this condition.

There is yet another crucial challenge or 'complication' with Lyme in relation to the goal of attaining a cure. This is misdiagnosis. Commonly, Lyme patients are diagnosed as having fibromyalgia, polymyositis, 'depression,' multiple sclerosis, ALS, schizophrenia, psychosis, and chronic fatigue syndrome. Lyme also specifically attacks the heart and nervous system. Thus, victims of Lyme and other tick bite diseases are also told that they have Bell's palsy, neuropathy, pericarditis, and cardiomyopathy, while tick bite diseases and Lyme as the cause are never considered.

A further aspect of Lyme, which confuses physicians, is its relapsing nature. Such a nature is typical of spirochetes. A person becomes relatively symptom free, and then it strikes again, devastating the individual. Spirochetes are notorious for causing such relapses. Other spirochetal diseases, which are known to cause relapsing disease include leptospirosis, syphilis, and tick-borne relapsing fever. Yet, in the United States, Canada, and Europe in particular Lyme should be suspected in any relapsing condition, especially if it is associated with the involvement of the joint and nervous systems.

The persistence of the infection is yet another aspect that bears emphasizing. A person takes a course of antibiotics and is regarded as 'cured.' The symptoms may well have improved and the main symptomology even reversed. Doctors deem the treatment a success. Yet, the Lyme spirochete still lurks in the body, merely transforming itself into a more well-hidden, chronic, and insidious form, one that escapes all immune surveillance.

Chapter Three

Biogerms on the Loose

It has already been established that prior to the 1970s there was no such condition as Lyme disease, at least none that was identified and confirmed—none that was confirmed in the medical literature. Then, how could such a devastating disease, which is so vast and widespread, be only a modern-day pandemic? It is a disease which is causing the devastation of the health of countless millions of people and it was never seen before, not in the 1960s or prior? How could it not have occurred in the previous decades and centuries, since ticks have existed long before the existence of civilized humankind?

Routinely, in that earlier era throughout the United States people got tick bites. In some cases they were bitten by multiple ticks, children included. Yet, whether adult or child prior to the 1960s and 1970s, no one was known to develop the constellation of symptoms as seen in Lyme disease, and, certainly, in the US there were no pocket outbreaks of the disease. It had struck suddenly, while primarily attacking children. Had this ever occurred before it would have been recorded and defined, plus an investigation would have been conducted, just as occurred in this original outbreak.

Definitively, there were no Lyme-like epidemics. Moreover, in all the medical textbooks published in the 1970s and prior no such precise syndrome was described.

This novel nature is supported by the circumstances surrounding its discovery. It was the work of a team of scientific investigators which finally confirmed it, climaxing in 1981 with the determination of the causative organism. There was no need for such a scientific investigation prior, because the condition didn't exist. At least that is what a reasonable assessment of the outbreak would conclude.

Orthodox sources beg to differ. The CDC-connected Website, American Lyme Disease Foundation, had this to say regarding the disease's origins:

> *Manifestations* of what we now call Lyme disease were first reported in medical literature in Europe in 1883. Over the years various clinical signs of this illness have been noted as separate medical conditions: acrodermatitis chronica atrophicans (ACA), lymphadenosis benigna cutis (LABC), erythema migrans (EM), and lymphocytic meningradiculitis (Bannwarth's syndrome). However, these diverse manifestations were not recognized as indicators of a single infectious illness until 1975, when Lyme disease was described following an *outbreak of apparent juvenile arthritis*, preceded by a rash, among residents of Lyme, Connecticut.

Overall, the write-up is an attempt to indicate that Lyme, as it is known today, has been with the world all along. Yet, that makes no sense. Surely, if this were a true, original disease, surely, it would havc been well defined in the medical literature, even if the cause was not known. Plus, as the write-up indicates there was no constellation of such symptoms ever seen before, especially in children.

Yet, despite attempts to suppress the origin of this pandemic, or even apologize for it, let us see what the CDC itself published in the major media:

> Monday, November 14, 2005
> UTSA opens new bioterrorism lab
> Associated Press
>
> SAN ANTONIO–A new research lab for bioterrorism opened Monday at the University of Texas at San Antonio.
>
> The $10.6 million Margaret Batts Tobin Laboratory Building will provide a 22,000-square-foot facility to study such diseases as anthrax, tularemia, cholera, lyme disease, desert valley fever and other parasitic and fungal diseases.
>
> The Centers for Disease Control and Prevention identified these diseases as *potential bioterrorism agents*. Fifteen university researchers make up the newly established South Texas Center for Emerging Infectious Diseases.
>
> Earlier this year, the researchers were awarded $9 million in federal funding for *bioterrorism research* conducted in a smaller lab on campus.

Potential bioterrorism agents, really? Who makes such bioterrorism agents, like anthrax and West Nile Virus, other than the mad scientists of the CDC and their fellow arch-corrupt military collaborators themselves?

It has already been made clear that the disease began as a spotty epidemic in Lyme, Connecticut. Why did it start there versus other areas? Connecticut is heavily wooded, yet so are dozens of other states such as New Jersey, Vermont, Rhode Island, Upstate New York, the Carolinas, Missouri, and others. It's not the woods that is the key factor. Nor is it naturally occurring ticks that have gone awry. In fact, the reason for this is far more insidious than most people realize.

Even so, it is realized that there are coincident factors. One of the main ones is the lack of traditional predators for mice, the main reservoir of the bacteria. An overpopulation of mice would lead to an excess number of ticks infested with the spirochete. Yet, could this alone lead to such a sudden epidemic in an isolated area? It is not plausible. The mice would surely have overpopulated a number of areas simultaneously.

The epidemic began in 1975 in a group of children living near each other. It only became recognized because of the astute observations of the mothers of such children. It was they who made researchers aware of what was happening, which was the fact that their children were developing rheumatoid arthritis-like illnesses. In fact, all the children had been diagnosed with rheumatoid arthritis. No such cluster of this condition in that age group in that area had ever before occurred.

The mothers knew there was something wrong. Children who had no prior history of joint disease were suddenly suffering from a crippling ailment. It made no sense, and it surely was unfathomable that multiple children in the same household were afflicted. The mothers approached medical professionals. 'Was there something in the environment that was making them sick, a toxin, a poison, or other,' they wondered? Too, the children who were so afflicted virtually all lived in heavily wooded areas. Quickly, the condition became known as Lyme disease.

In a sense the name is a misnomer. The disease should be renamed based upon the cause and bacteriology. It would be better to call it Tick-Based BioWarefare Spirochetal Disease than Lyme. Or, at least it should be deemed Tick-Based Spirochetal Disease. In fact, without the spirochete there would be no such condition. Therefore, rather than a geographical issue—'Lyme' disease—this is an infectious condition, and all the symptoms are due to infection.

While the vast majority of cases of Lyme are the result of tick bites there are other modes of transmission. It is believed that in some cases mosquitoes are the vectors. Too, it has been confirmed that some people develop the disease as a result of blood transfusion and also through intrauterine transfer. It all originates, though, not from ticks but, rather, from lower animals. Infected ticks acquire the Lyme spirochete from biting various animals, notably rodents. In fact, mice, rats, shrews, and other animals of the rodent family, such as ground squirrels, are the primary source of this potentially deadly pathogen.

Ticks are bloodsuckers. So, whatever is in the blood of its victims it will acquire. The vile ticks then breed the germ, carrying it in their stomachs. They merely inject it into any victim of their bites, at which time the spirochete begins the process of invading the body. The invasion begins locally, that is at the site of the bite, proceeding systemically to the blood, lymph, and, ultimately, internal organs.

The tick responsible for Lyme usually attacks people through its stealthiest form, the mere immature nymph. The bloodthirsty nymph is no bigger than the head of a pin. It's as if its entire purpose is to operate via disguise. Virtually no one sees it when it does its dastardly deed, since it is some 100 times tinier than the adult form. Only on rare occasions will it be seen in time to kill it before it infects. Therefore, most victims have no idea they have been bitten or that they actually have a tick on while the disease is being transmitted. They may miss it even after carefully inspecting the body for the presence of ticks. Furthermore, larger ticks can be felt as they crawl up the body. With the nymph form of the deer tick people usually do not feel it crawling or sense its presence.

All this makes Lyme disease a category of its own. In fact, there is virtually no other disease like it. A person is in fine health, then, suddenly succumbs to a potentially deadly disease and has no idea what is the cause.

Once it fully infects the body, it is too late. The infection becomes established in the bloodstream and internal organs, after which the hideous disease begins its attack.

One of the most treacherous infectious diseases known even with the most potent medicines, orthodox or natural, Lyme is not easy to eradicate. The infectious agent gains residence deep within the body, where it multiplies, causing potentially life-threatening disease. A major effort must be made to purge it. If not, it may recur, and the cycle could be endless.

For a total cure to be achieved all traces of the Lyme spirochete must be purged from the body. This must be done at all costs, that is in order for normal, good health to return.

Drugs can't entirely do this. The bacteria will mutate, altering themselves into even stealthier forms. Only natural germicides can do so. Too, only nature can be relied upon to fully support the body's health, that is support and strengthen the immune system, so it can fight back against this disease. This is through the intake of unprocessed, natural-source spice extracts, herbal supplements, wild, raw purging agents, and also health-giving, vitalizing foods.

Despite this, there is no denying the value of antibiotics in this disease. Too, antibiotics are a kind of natural cure. They are an exception in the realm of the largely synthetic drugs. Thus, the intake of such drugs may be necessary in Lyme. Even so, here, natural options to antibiotics are offered for those who choose this type of therapy—and for those who may be ultra-sensitive to the toxicity of antibiotics.

Even so, is it not unfathomable? The world has become an exceedingly dangerous place to live. Even in non-tropical regions, like the United States and Europe, it is possible to contract a life-threatening disease merely through no extraordinary incident, like cutting wood, playing in a area of tall grass or woods, or picnicking in the forest. A hunting or fishing trip or, perhaps, an outing to pick wild herbs or berries may result in the contraction of a tick-based disease.

That forest seems peaceful enough. A walk through the forest or a bit of investigation into the woods; who would deem this dangerous, that is until the existence of Lyme was known? Direly, it is now known that lurking in the midst of the forests is a treachery that is more dangerous than the fiercest, most dangerous of all wild beasts.

Worldwide, in terms of the contraction of diseases and disabilities ticks are among the most dangerous of all insects, secondary only to mosquitos. No one wants to be bitten by a tick: how vile. These insects are among the most wretched, darkest of all, existing in the most vile of all states: as parasites of rodents. When they bite humans, they give these humans the rodent germs. By no means have all the various germs living in rodent blood been identified, as well as various germs from whatever animals they are in contact with, including dogs and cats. *Borrelia burgdorferi,* anaplasma, rickettsia (ehrlichia and others), and babesia are all rodent-based.

On every continent there are ticks which readily attack and infect humans. Dozens of syndromes caused by such tick bites are now documented. Lyme, though, is among the most devastating of all diseases transmitted by ticks. It is pervasive in North America, especially in the US's upper northeastern coastal and upper midwestern states.

Chapter Four

Conspiracy to Kill

It has already been established that prior to the 1970s there was no such condition as Lyme disease. As a natural disease it is not plausible that it could arrive from virtually nowhere, as if descending from outer space. The lack of its description in the US-based medical literature alone is a cause for suspicion. This is highly significant, since even the rarest of diseases are well described. Thus, for the widespread development of such a novel syndrome there had to be a specific, traceable origin. Since it occurred in a cluster, it had to be associated with a discoverable element. Moreover, that element pointed to human meddling.

Since there have always been ticks and tick bites, how could such a debilitating and potentially deadly disease arise spontaneously? Surely, with the panorama of symptoms seen in Lyme, especially its initial presentation as single joint disease, along with a rash, in many instances someone would have noticed it. Someone in the medical or research community would have made note of it, even publishing an article about it as a potentially new condition.

Was it, then, the breakdown of the immune system in modern humans that allowed the tick-transmitted germ to overpopulate and thus cause the disease? Did pollution play a predominant role? Was there a poison in the soil or environment particular to that region alone? Was it poor nutrition that was a key element, that is gross or moderate nutritional deficiency in the body, making the people who acquired it more vulnerable? Is it the trend of living near wooded areas that is responsible? Incredibly, there is sufficient evidence to regard the origin as far more insidious than these, although surely such issues play a role. Lyme is by all the evidence a man-made condition, specifically the result of the bioengineering of novel germs.

Could it really be the case? Is there actual proof that the origin of the disease is an experiment that went awry? Even more diabolical was it released intentionally, that is was it meant to be an experiment on humans to see if they would contract the disease? Then, could all the misery and suffering caused by Lyme have been prevented? Could it be that it never was a naturally occurring disease at all?

If it can be proven that it is a man-made condition, surely those who are responsible would be held accountable. The immense harm they have caused; surely, they would be identified and brought down on charges for the devastation they have wrought, including the ruination of the health of countless millions of people and also the outright killing of people. Absolutely, they would be dealt with according to the law of the land. Murder charges against the originators of the lab and the mad scientists they employed, the ones responsible for the spread of Lyme, would be brought to bear. Finally, there would be divine justice. Yet, is it even possible?

In fact, no such justice will ever occur, at least not on this planet. This is despite the fact that the real source of the Lyme pandemic can be readily proven. Even the "who," that is who specifically is responsible, can be demonstrated.

Plum Island: corruption to the extreme

The source of the Lyme pandemic cannot be mere natural spread or encroachment of modern humans upon the wilderness. Rather, it is a consequence of human meddling. Lyme disease is directly tied to the activities of a bioweapons lab located just off America's shores. Found on Plum Island, New York, the lab is closest in proximity to Connecticut, whose shores are a mere 10 miles from the facility.

A proven bioweapons research lab, the operations of the Plum Island facility were always top secret. No one could readily determine precisely what the scientists and their military cohorts were doing. At first it was reportedly a top secret military facility, later to be converted to a so-called veterinarian research lab.

It is now shuttered. No one can gain access to it, no journalist and no independent investigator.

It is no wonder. The connection of the lab to Lyme disease is seemingly direct and absolute. The facility was heavily involved in research on various biological agents: potentially deadly germs, which were specially cultured for their devastating effects. The purpose was to use such germs as agents in the battlefield. For these military associated scientists the challenge was how to deliver the germ load to the 'enemy' while not causing infection of the 'good guys.' Dropping germs in the battlefield in general was deemed too risky. For instance, in close battle the wind could carry the deployed germs in an undesirable direction, right upon Western forces.

There had to be a more controlled, direct way to deliver the infectious disease payload to the purported target. The answer was found, so it was believed, through biting insects. The purpose was to infect the insects with disease-causing germs and then use them on the battlefield as transporting agents to infect the 'enemy' specifically.

These insects are known as vectors. A vector is defined as "an organism, typically a biting insect (or tick), which transmits a disease or parasite..."

It is now known definitively that the labs of this island did a vast amount of research on such vectors. Researchers would infect ticks and mosquitos with a variety of germs and then evaluate them to see if they could transmit those infections. No wonder both Lyme disease and West Nile virus broke out, initially, in both cases in regions of close proximity to the island.

Let there be no doubt about it human meddling is responsible for the outbreaks of such diseases, the tick spirochete epidemic occurring originally in Connecticut, while West Nile broke out in New York State. It is these two states which are closest to the biogerm-producing facility. It is a certainty that the operators of the lab infected both mosquitoes and ticks with disease-causing agents. Then, they unleashed these infected insects into the environment. The outbreaks of both Lyme and West Nile were covered-up, so no one would realize the source.

Yet, what were they thinking, if they ever gave thought at all to their actions? How could they possibly control the ultimate results of what they were doing? They truly were/are mad scientists, that is mad enough to refuse to consider the consequences of their acts. The risks were obviously never considered. It was all overridden by the zealous desire to be superior, to prevail against any perceived enemy at any expense, even the expense of the destruction of the local population.

So, the research went on. Experiments were performed. Infected mosquitos and ticks were released. If as a result of such research it could be determined that the insects could transmit the disease to humans, the goal would be achieved. Now, it was planned, the infected vectors would be produced in quantity. Bombs and artillery shells tainted with such biogerm-infested vectors would be produced. These bombs and shells would then be dropped and/or lobbed upon the enemy soldiers, or at least that was the plot at hand.

The purpose wasn't necessarily to kill the enemy outright. Rather, it was to weaken a fighting force to such a degree that it would be rendered useless. Then, the righteous armies would attack these weakened forces, destroying them in vast numbers.

What a miserable goal it was and what a vile, wretched plot—in fact, such perpetrators should be brought down on murder charges. Even more vile is the consequences, which is the fact that instead of such treachery being committed on the battlefield it was heaped instead upon the general population, people all over the world. Virtually all such people, victims of Lyme, are, apparently, victims of Plum Island research.

Even so, for those who might find such words dubious let it be known that the hierarchy of the lab has admitted to the same. According to the facility's ex-director Jerry Callis "Plum Island *experimented with ticks*." Some of those experiments included *open air tests*, meaning the ticks were *released into the environment*. In many respects Plum Island was a tick disease research center. Therefore, the connection is clear. The ticks harboring the *Borrelia burgdorferi* and which caused the initial outbreak were creations of Plum Island researchers. It's hard to call them researchers. Zealots or fanatics would be better terms. They created a true pandora's box situation. Once it was out of that 'box,' actually, containment, the unknown truly did occur, which was the wreaking of vast havoc on this world.

Operation Paperclip: CIA's mad scientists and more

Upon further analysis the plot thickens. The research on such vectors infamously had its roots in Nazi Germany. Nazi, actually, Ashkenazi, agents involved in such investigations were brought to the United States under the CIA-instituted program known as Operation Paperclip.

Says Barbara J. Andrews, Editor-in-Chief, of TheDogPress.com:

> The nefarious history of Plum Island began after World War II, when Erich Traub, a German biological warfare expert, joined the team. Our government learned of the German penchant for bio-weapons technology through defectors.

Significantly, Traub operated a germ warfare lab in the Baltic Sea. The criminal mind was recruited by factions within the US government to lead the research at the island facility.

How could this be possible? Was the war even real? Clearly, powerful elements of the US government were directly collaborating with the supposed enemy. Traub was Heinrich Himmler's former Racial and Biological Chemical Warfare scientist. Yet, incredibly, simultaneously he worked secretly for the US Naval Medical Research Institute and the early elements of the CIA? The fact is, covertly, Traub was brought to the U.S. during Operation Paperclip along with *2000 other Nazis*. The organizers of this plot were directors of the OSS and CIA, that is America's spy agencies.

In Nazi Germany Traub's expertise included infecting mosquitos and ticks with biological agents. Notes Andrews, according to the USDA there were "virus outbreaks, biological meltdowns, infected workers..." There was also the admitted release of germ-tainted raw waste into Long Island Sound. Importantly, the documents also revealed "*experimental tick colonies*" were bred for the purpose of '*spreading'* disease here.

The key word is experimental. At a militarized lab what would they be experimenting on? They surely weren't growing ticks as merely a biology experiment. Regardless, who in the world would seek to grow their own ticks? Clearly, the insects were produced for nefarious purposes, and the experimental part was the purposeful infection of such ticks with potentially deadly germs, including *Borrelia burgdorferi.*

Here is another key proving the conspiracy. The USDA document describing the tick experiments was dated 1975, *the same year Lyme broke out just off the shores of Connecticut.*

One germ that was admittedly infected into the ticks is the well-published experimental pathogen, *Mycoplasma fermentans*. This germ is fully a man-made mutant, to such a degree that a patent is held on it as a semi-synthetic pathogen. As a battlefield germ *Mycoplasma fermentans* is an extremely powerful weakening agent. This pathogen is commonly found in the bloodstream of Lyme disease victims.

Yet, as a source of Lyme, too, the documentation is forthcoming, even though the former lab operators offer nothing other than denials. In 2002 it was the highly regarded *Journal of Degenerative Diseases* that made the connection. In this journal it was revealed that the former War Department research lab *is* the source of Lyme disease. At the time of the article it was made clear that Plum Island had identified itself as an "animal research lab." What the article did make clear is that the mycoplasma agent found in Lyme patients is the "same pathogen (*Mycoplasma fermentans*) found in Gulf War Illness, fibromyalgia, and chronic fatigue syndrome" patients.

As mentioned previously the proximity gives evidence of a biogerm connection. Plum Island is exceedingly close to heavily inhabited coastal regions. It sits on Long Island Sound, with one end pointing directly towards the Connecticut coast, the other toward Long Island's North Fork.

Is this not treacherous to the extreme? Life is difficult enough with all the health challenges people face without adding to the burden, without this human race having to endure the tyranny of man-made infections.

The "experimental" method used by Traub and his coterie of mad scientists was devious to the extreme. Biological agents were cultured and altered to the desired point, largely with the purpose of making them more vigorous as disease causing agents. Then, these cultured, if not novel, germs were infected into ticks and mosquitoes. Next, as a further element of the experiment these tainted insects were released into the environment.

Apparently, on the island they were released for the purpose of infecting the local or migrating animals. The next step was that the animals were 'monitored' to see if they became overcome with the desired disease.

Then, the incredible occurred. The germ in the form of the tick bioweapon began attacking the general public. It was the people at-large who became the victims of this biowarfare plot, not some mysterious presumed enemy. It was they who were exclusively weakened, denuded, and corrupted, even killed. It was and is they who have been turned into the enemy.

It's not that tick bites have ever been a minor issue. For instance, Rocky Mountain Spotted Fever, caused by a rickettsial germ, is commonly fatal. It's just that it has always been a regional disease. Lyme is global. The damage done by the US-based bioweapons research lab is incalculable. All that can be done, now, is to help the sufferers as much as possible and also to do all that is possible to prevent the disease.

Eventually, the ticks made their way to the continent, Long Island and Connecticut apparently being infested first. Whether or not the ticks were purposely released on the mainland is unknown. A likely mechanism is that they became attached to birds, which then delivered them to the coastal regions. This could explain their concentration in the woods of Connecticut, Long Island, New Jersey, Pennsylvania, and more. Even so, a purposeful release cannot be ruled out. It had been done before, notoriously by the CIA and U.S. Military, among others.

Rodents could also have been the source, as they are capable of swimming such a distance. A ten mile swim for them from Plum Island to the shores of Connecticut is a minor trip. The tick-infested rodents and/or birds, then, delivered their deadly cargo to the area, from which higher mammals became infected, including deer, dogs, and humans. Regions in New York State, New Jersey, and Connecticut quickly became overrun. From there it spread nationally then, ultimately, internationally. It is now a permanent source of disease, thanks exclusively to human corruption.

Who would know?

It bears repeating. When that aggregation of cases occurred in Lyme, Connecticut, the disease baffled physicians. None of the physicians who saw the cases pinned it on the actual cause, which is an infection from tick bites. This fact would tend to confirm Plum Island as the source of the epidemic versus a naturally occurring cause.

No wonder the doctors were clueless. The constellation of symptoms of this condition had never before been seen. There had never been a cluster of such an outbreak previously, where children in particular were afflicted with a rheumatoid arthritis-like disease. It all started out in a way, which became a classical case of epidemiological discovery. As described by D. R. Snydman in his essay, "Principles of Epidemiology," which is actually a chapter in the book, *Mechanisms of Microbial Disease*, it all started out in the classical way of a disease unknown and/or newly discovered. This was when the Department of Health of Connecticut received "separate phone calls from two mothers living on rural roads in the towns of Lyme and Old Lyme." What the mothers reported was dire, which was the fact that "*several children in their households and the neighborhood had what appeared to be arthritis*."

This, then, represents none other than hard proof of the fraud. It was a clear and categorical outbreak of a disease never before known. Children do not suddenly develop arthritis primarily presenting as single joint disease—that is they never do so in pocket outbreaks, not in the history of American medicine. Furthermore, if there is the development of such a condition in a family, it afflicts only one child, not multiples of them.

Even so, in the 1970s ticks along the East Coast didn't suddenly and miraculously become so pathological. They were inoculated maliciously for this purpose, which was to transmit crippling diseases.

While it might be difficult for some people to fathom, there is seemingly no other possibility. Clearly, the Plum Island corrupt ones created this monster, possibly as a kind of weaponized syphilis. Of note, it should be realized that the latter also presents as acutely damaged and/or swollen single joint disease.

They were under attack. These were previously normal children. Vital, healthy—and highly mobile—they suddenly become afflicted with crippling joint conditions? Moreover, it is the children, not the adults? Too, it happens to multiple children in the same household? Plus, these are virtually all families living in a rural setting near woods. Furthermore, there are dogs in association, while the children have a history of playing in the woods. Moreover, it all occurs coincident with tick-vector research on that notorious island a mere 10 miles from Lyme. The epidemiology leads not merely to tick bites but also to Plum Island as the source of the highly pathogenic—and pathological—germ.

Despite this, to certain scientific minds it did seem sufficiently bizarre. Unlike the local physicians who had treated the cases, the epidemiologists working for the state decided that this was a novel condition. People had lived in that area for decades, and none of them developed any such condition, surely not the children. Therefore, they deemed, it warranted further investigation.

The state looked in depth at the cluster of childhood cases. Here is what they found. In all cases there was arthritis, but it was not the standard kind seen in the elderly. This was, in fact, a bizarre type, which fits precisely the history and presentation of infective arthritis. Almost everyone presented, initially, with a single joint, which became unexplainably swollen. It was always a large joint, like a knee, ankle, elbow, shoulder, or other, just as in its sister disease syphilis. The swelling largely incapacitated the victims and thus was a cause for alarm among the parents. Once again, this is the standard presentation for acute bacterial infection of the body. Other bacterial agents which present as single joint disease include gonococcal infection and relapsing spirochetal fever.

It must be emphasized that this initial presentation of single joint arthritis was universal in all the victims. It cannot be described often enough. That's because it is the key to the diagnosis of Lyme, then and now. In the original outbreak the single joint presentation put the investigators on the right track. It led to the consideration by the researchers of the existence of an infectious agent. There was another common finding in many of the sufferers. This was a bizarre, never-before-experienced oval rash. The rash was of fairly large size. Sometimes, it would recur, either in the same place or elsewhere on the body. In some cases the rash disappeared completely. Such a large rash associated with single joint swelling and/or arthritis was clearly a new finding for East Coast physicians. They had no idea what they were dealing with and did not on their own determine the cause.

This is not to say that infectious tick-borne spirochetes had never occurred before. Yet, they had never occurred in such severity, with such symptoms and disability and/or in clustered outbreaks in children.

The association of the disease with the activities on Plum Island is clear. Moreover, the biogerm worked just as advertised. It incapacitated its victims. Later, it would become known that in some cases it killed them.

Chapter Five

Lab Freaks and Bizarre Yeasts

For the secretive facility 1975 was a year of extensive, and now fully admitted, tick vector research. To survive all germs must feed. Thus, in order to maintain the colonies the animals were experimentally infected by the ticks. The Lyme bacteria can only survive within living animal tissue. Regarding this germ wretched as it seems its preferred foods appear to be skin tissue, joint tissue, and nervous system tissue. In this regard it will be recalled that the spirochete is known as a "corkscrew pathogen." The purpose of such an anatomy and physiology relates to its feeding propensity. It bores into tissue, so it can eat it. Unopposed, what is the result? It will be nothing but agonizing misery, as the spirochetes multiply, consume, and, consequently, destroy.

After injection by the tick, rapidly, there develops countless billions of such pathogens in the body, attacking tissues, destroying cells. The death of the cells is known medically as apoptosis. The cells essentially implode. White blood cells attempt to purge the spirochete, yet because of its capacities to evade the immune system it attacks and decimates these protective cells, too. How dire it is, formerly healthy cells being killed off by a germ derived from a biting insect.

Therefore, with all the powers that are conceivable the Lyme spirochete must be opposed. It must be attacked and destroyed, just as it attacks and destroys. Whether drugs or natural complexes all the most potent remedies available must be launched against it. Thus, it must be stopped in its tracks, rather, obliterated.

In chronic Lyme any attempts to destroy the pathogenic culprits have largely failed. In this regard studies have shown that even after long-term antibiotic therapy the Lyme spirochete survives and, in fact, often thrives extensively. Thus, to some degree this condition is regarded by the medical profession as incurable, especially in those cases which prove refractory to antibiotics. There is no accepted belief that herbal medicines are of value. Claims demonstrating their value are often completely dismissed. Thus, other than the use of various drugs the attitude is "nothing can be done."

No doubt, certain antibiotics do kill the Lyme bacillus or at least do so temporarily. Yet, these antibiotics are impotent versus a number of co-infection agents, particularly viruses and protozoans. Even for primary, acute Lyme the antibiotics may prove inadequate, failing miserably. Even so, such failures are rarely reported in the medical literature, where the claim is that drug therapy is 90% effective in achieving a cure. That claim, though, is now heavily disputed.

Regarding alternative medicine such negativity must be disregarded. As will be demonstrated here for the vast majority of cases of this disease, whether acute or chronic, natural medicines are the answer. While it is a challenge with Lyme the body can be healed and the infection eliminated. Once such infection is purged from the tissues, the symptoms will largely disappear. The sufferer must never give up. Moreover, in addition to any medical therapy natural medicines should also be vigorously used. There is no harm in using them together. Too, for those who choose it is possible to rely on natural cures preferentially as the main source of treatment. In particular, oil of wild oregano in super-strength form and also the dessicated, encapsulated spice oils—oils of wild oregano and sage, along with cumin and cinnamon oils—aggressively kill the spirochete.

In my case the approach was to use exclusively natural cures, relying mainly on a high strength version of the wild oil of oregano, along with the multiple spice dried oil capsules, to avoid the potential danger of drugs. This danger includes the side effects of candida overgrowth as well as the potential for liver and kidney toxicity.

Candida albicans: a cause of Lyme or a side-effect?

In many instances the notorious yeast *Candida albicans* plays a significant role in Lyme disease. The yeast/fungus is a more prominent factor in the event of the overuse of antibiotics, which is surely the case in countless Lyme victims.

A single course of antibiotics can lead to candida infection. What, then, results from the taking of such drugs for a month or longer? There are people with this condition who have taken antibiotics for several months and up to a year. All such people have systemic candida overload.

Antibiotic-induced candida growth is noxious. Normally, this yeast is kept in check by the healthy bacteria, that is the probiotics. The yeast is a normal organism, known as a commensal. Yet, typically, it only accounts for a mere three percent of the gut flora population. It is the balance of all such germs that counts, that is for the maintenance of ideal health.

Antibiotics drastically change that. By systematically wiping out the gut flora they create a void. Essentially, an entire component of the immune system has been abolished through this toxicity. This is highly dangerous, because of the fact that these drugs do not kill *Candida albicans* and other yeasts. Therefore, these yeasts fill in the gap, overpopulating the intestinal tract. Moreover, they do so in an aggressive, destructive way.

Of the various potential gut pathogens candida is highly novel. In research conducted at the University of Iowa it was determined that when a variety of germs were blasted with X-rays, it was this yeast which best survived, mutating into dozens of new forms. Candida does all that it can to survive, altering itself upon exposure to stress. Antibiotics 'stress' the candida by attacking its cell wall. Thus, in its infinite wisdom the pathogen compensates, transforming itself into a new entity. Essentially, the germ re-makes itself without a cell wall, the new yeast being appropriately known as cell wall deficient. This form of candida is highly toxic. Yet, it succumbs to the powers of wild spice oils, which, essentially, burn it to death.

Another type of candida is the mycelial form. The mycelia are a kind of invasive tentacle created by the fungus to bore into the tissues. As a result of the overgrowth of this form great inflammation is caused in the tissues, especially the cell linings of the organs, known as the mucous membranes. This form of candida overgrowth is known medically as mucocutaneous candidiasis, in other words, mucous membrane candida infection.

In such infection a wide range of mucous membranes may be involved. The membranes that suffer candida overgrowth as a result of the overuse of antibiotics include those lining the gut, the main area of attack, but also those which line the mouth, sinus cavities, bronchial tubes, kidneys, bladder, urethra, prostate, uterus, fallopian tubes, and vaginal tract. All such membrane linings can become extensively inflamed as a result of antibiotic toxicity. Essentially, it is a form of yeast thrush of these regions, one that is manifested by in the case of antibiotic overuse deep-seated infestation.

The symptoms of candida overgrowth are diverse and vast. Many of the signs and symptoms are a result of toxins produced by the yeast as well as the irritation/inflammation resulting from its invasive capacities. Usually, no doctor recognizes these symptoms as being caused by the yeast. Such symptoms include the following:

- sore, inflamed mouth and/or tongue
- burning tongue
- itchy ears
- itching of the skin
- outbreaks of eczema and/or psoriasis
- chronic sore throat
- heartburn
- chronic bladder disorders
- vaginitis or thrush
- vaginal discharge
- abdominal cramps
- PMS
- ovarian cysts
- prostate inflammation
- mental fogginess
- fatigue
- fibromyalgia-like symptoms
- cold hands and feet
- sinus disorders
- bronchial disorders and/or asthma

- flu-like syndrome
- extreme sensitivity to fumes and chemicals
- cravings for sugar or sweets
- cravings for alcohol, especially wine and beer
- chronic constipation
- alternating constipation and diarrhea
- spastic colon and/or irritable bowel syndrome

The degree of symptoms resulting from candida infestation is vast. This is why it is known as the great mimicker. The mutated, invasive candida must be destroyed for symptoms to be alleviated and normal function to return.

Candida plus Lyme surely complicates issues. This may explain the refractory nature of many chronic Lyme disease cases, the ones that fail to respond to orthodox therapy. This is especially true of those who have been treated with a number of courses of antibiotics. Candida infestation in particular may account for those who actually worsen with drug therapy.

This demonstrates, once again, the invaluable nature of spice oil extracts. These extracts are highly potent not only against the Lyme bacillus but also against candida. In fact, they have a great potency against all yeasts and molds, which they categorically kill. Even so, as mentioned previously there is a caveat. It is the potential negative effects against the good bacteria, especially in high doses. Yet, the spice oils do not cause the type of widespread toxicity, as caused by antibiotics, where there is the creation of mutated, invasive forms of this pathogen. Therefore, they are preferable for prolonged intake in the case of Lyme and/or chronic Lyme versus antibiotics. At least the spice oils should be taken adjunctively with these drugs. In all such cases, whether taking the drugs alone, the oil of wild oregano as the primary therapy, or the two together, probiotic supplements should be consumed. So should there be a heavy intake of foods rich in healthy bacteria, including high-grade whole food yogurt, quark, kefir, and sauerkraut.

Candida infestation is a major dilemma in the battle against Lyme. The existence of such yeast overgrowth has great suppressive effects against the immune system. Too, the toxins produced as a result of the excessive numbers of candida also depress immune health. Thus, it must be cleansed from the body. Fortunately, any effort at doing so simultaneously purges the Lyme and co-infection agents.

Protocol for candida yeast cleansing/purging

- oil of wild oregano (edible form, mountain-grown): 10 or more drops twice daily
- multiple spice dessicated (dry) capsules or sublingual drops: if capsules, two twice daily with meals: if oil, 20 drops twice daily with meals
- whole, crude wild oregano complex plus *Rhus coriaria*, garlic, and onion: 3 or more capsules twice daily
- healthy bacterial supplement (Ecologic 500 or another of similar quality): heaping teaspoonful at night in warm water (or as capsules,whatever is available)

Note: in the event of deep-seated yeast infestation in the colon there is a special type of wild oregano, multiple spice-based formula that is available. This formula consists of oils of wild oregano, sage, and bay leaf, along with cumin oil, emulsified in bee's wax. What an ideal formula it is, since the bee's wax causes the wild oregano and other spice oil medicines to be gently yet effectively delivered into the lower reaches of the intestines, that is the lower small intestine, the colon, and the rectum. For moderate candida overgrowth take two twice daily and for severe, three or more twice daily.

Allow 30 to 90 days of spice oil therapy to fully purge the fungus from the tissues. The key is to stay the course, taking the spice oil regimen at least twice daily. In some cases it may take up to six months to fully purge all traces of the yeast from the tissues. For extreme cases up to six months or even a year of such therapy may be necessary.

There are those who claim, including medical professionals, that the oregano oil/spice oil therapy should be staggered, that it should be stopped and other therapies applied. Some of these individuals, notably naturopathic therapists, add: "Oregano oil should not be taken for a long course; it's toxic." In this they are categorically wrong. In fact, it is dangerous to start and stop such therapy. The wild oregano oil must be used continuously until the eradication is achieved, that is if it is the truly wild-growing edible spice-based variety—and this could be nowhere more true than regarding candida and Lyme.

In fact, it is the failure to use the treatment for a sufficient amount of time that is the issue. As demonstrated by research conducted at Georgetown University if the treatment course is too short, the fungus will return. This is why it is necessary to take the therapy for a minimum of one or two months. Plus, for optimal results the usage should be daily during this period of time. Furthermore, regarding the original, true wild oregano oil and multiple spice complex even with daily use there is no such toxicity, even with prolonged doses. Rather, as a rule as a result of the vigorous intake of such spice oils the function of the detoxification organs, the liver and the kidneys, improves.

Even so, there are certain moderate-to-minor issues which must be discussed. This includes the potential for gastric irritation from spice oils, especially the multiple spice dessicated formula. In such a case it is advisable to take such a formula with meals. Too, there can be so-called die-off, where a person seemingly gets worse before feeling better. This is always temporary and is generally reversed by actually increasing the dose rather than decreasing it. As always, for those with sensitive systems take any new supplement to tolerance. Die-off symptoms are often relieved through the intake of wild oregano/*Rhus coriaria* capsules.

Yet, regarding the liver and the kidneys how could such powerful spice oils actually improve the function of these organs? It is a result of their purging power, that is their ability to purge dangerous pathogens from the body, including those which may infect the organs of detoxification. Moreover, it is the pathogens which cause stress upon the body, so their removal is a positive issue, reducing the toxic burden on the liver, kidneys, and other organs. It is well established, for instance, that fungal invaders, like *Candida albicans*, cause significant toxicity to the organs, largely through the production of mycotoxins. Oil of wild oregano, as well as oils of cumin, sage, bay leaf, and cinnamon, destroy such toxins.

Too, spice oils are potent antioxidants. For instance, oil of wild oregano is some 100 times more potent in the quenching of free radicals than blueberry. Oil of clove is some 300 times more powerful than this fruit, while cumin oil is nearly 80 times as potent. Thus, the intake of such food-grade spice oils actually protects the organs from damage, never damaging them. Rather clinical tests on humans have demonstrated an improvement in kidney and liver function through the intake of such oils, that is the edible types as found in the wild high-mountain-source material, the whole, crude wild herb, the wild juice of oregano, and the multiple spice complex dessicated oil capsules.

Note: this degree of exceptional safety is true of the edible, wild spice oil supplements made by North American Herb & Spice. Do not accept cheap imitations made with Spanish thyme, Moroccan oregano, *Origanum vulgare*, and/or Mexican sage.

Chapter Six

Danger in the Woods

It was a near death experience that was the motivation for the writing of these words. This was in regard to a happening in the Wisconsin woods. Actually, it all occurred on a work project.

The project involved the aggressive picking of a wild berry. It was the wild black raspberry which was being sought, which is relatively rare to find in large patches and also tedious to pick. Yet, it is worth the effort, since this wild berry is one of the most potent anti-tumor berries known in America.

For the making of a raw extract there was a deficiency of the raw material and thus a need to hunt more down. No one else would seemingly do it. Thus, I, along with a small crew, went into the wild Wisconsin woods and fields to do the picking.

The berries were to be picked, then, while in a fresh, raw state taken immediately back to the facility. There, the raw liquor would be extracted through cold-pressing. It would then be preserved raw for use as a natural medicine as sublingual drops.

It is all hand-done, and such extracts are quite rare, especially in regard to wild berries. Finding patches of wild black raspberries of sufficient size to meet the demand is no easy project. Routinely, these patches are found in the most remote areas conceivable, away from human invasion—precisely the areas inhabited by wild creatures, particularly deer, wild predators, rodents, and more.

The grass was tall, and the woods scrubby, which is ideal tick territory. There were oak trees in the area, a favorite haunt of these creatures. It even looked dangerous and to a degree corrupt, although it was uninhabited and far away from human influence. Thus, the necessary precautions were taken. For several days the picking went on. White disposable hazmat-style suits were used. The socks were pulled over the pant legs. A natural-source repellant spray was applied made from oils of wild bay leaf, lavender, and oregano, along with clove oil (Herbal Tick-X).

The berry region was seemingly picked in-full, without incident. Throughout this time no ticks were seen. Then, as the lead picker I decided to go out one more time on my own. As I had seen no ticks in this last adventure, no precautions were taken. It was a rather hot day, and the suit was a bit suffocating. No suit was worn; no spray was applied. This proved to be disastrous.

It was surely preventable. A single omission, a single element of neglect, led to a near fatal catastrophe. That preventive precaution, of drawing up the socks over the pant legs has always been so valuable. It prevents stealth attacks by ticks in unseen areas. It was nearly the end of the summer. "The tick season seems to be over, " I thought. Yet, it was not so.

Within a week a great disaster occurred. A sickness struck that was difficult to understand. There was sudden exhaustion. The head was pounding, the neck stiff. Bizarre sensations were felt in the spine, as if it was full. It felt as if the head was exploding. In my head, in fact, there was mind-bending pain. It felt, too, as if I was burning up, and, in particular, there was a sensation as if the skin was on fire. "What in the world is going on? Why can't I function? Why do I feel like I am burning alive?" It must be admitted that to a degree there was a sense of panic. "Whatever this is, will I live or die?" It truly was that dire.

Yet, "What was causing the body to feel as if it was exploding?" I wondered. "Wait a minute, I feel something truly bizarre on my back. It's an unexplainable burning sensation, extremely irritating. "What is it?" Then, I turned around and looked in the mirror. What a shock it was. There was a large bull's eye rash, oval in shape. It was the size of a small, flattened football and traversed most of the length of my mid-to lower back.

"Oh my God," I said, "I've contracted Lyme disease—so that's what this is all about." Moreover, it was clear that it was a severe case and that it was not caught sufficiently early, that is early enough to quickly reverse the symptoms.

The shocking decline in health dramatically continued. It felt as if the entire body was exploding. The rash area, too, was exceedingly uncomfortable. "What was going on in the spinal column, neck, and head?" They felt so full, as if they were going to explode. The head felt full, too, as if there was a bomb about to go off in it.

There was also a fullness in the inguinal area as well as the lateral aspect of the neck. "My lymph glands are swollen," I realized. "It is all over my body."

It was a desperate situation. It was clear that the Lyme bacillus, the spirochete *Borrelia burgdorferi,* was attacking my entire system. "What is a person to do? I don't want to go on the standard treatment." With my history of candida I was afraid it would come raging back, as antibiotics kill the normal flora, allowing the yeast to gain a foothold. Additionally, despite the value of antibiotics in Lyme there are potential side effects in the realm of organ toxicity, including liver and kidney toxicity as well as in the case of tetracyclines a poisonous action on the immune and nervous systems.

"I must use natural antibacterial substances, natural antiseptics despite the dire nature of my condition," I thought. Thus, without hesitation I turned to the oil of oregano and other wild oregano/spice derivatives such as the juice of wild oregano and the multiple spice dried oil complex.

In fact, without the natural spice oil extracts with their potent germicidal—and anti-spirochetal powers—there is no hope for the aggressive reversal of disease, that is for those who seek a natural-source treatment. Antibiotics alone are incapable of curing the majority of cases of Lyme, particularly in cases where the onset is not recognized until well after the infestation occurred.

Regardless, the situation was corrupt—the spinal fullness and stiffness, the fullness in the head, the headaches, and the sensation that my entire head and spine were about to explode. The issue was clear. I had developed a potentially fatal condition known as neuroborreliosis.

Apparently, it was meant to be. Perhaps, it was so this book would be written. It was so an example could be made, paving the way for new discoveries, various means by which Lyme could be cured without pharmaceutical drugs or in concert with them. Could it be that this discovery was necessary in order to aid the endless suffering of Lyme patients, desperate victims of a conspiracy against modern humanity? If so, then, the pain and agony was worth it, revealing new knowledge, new discoveries, for the sake of others.

Too, antibiotics would have likely caused an improvement in the condition, although they would have brought on the dreaded candidiasis condition. Yet, there was no guarantee of it. Even with full medical treatment Lyme often persists, with some 40% of cases failing to respond.

One of the other risks of long-term antibiotic therapy is the development of mutated bacteria, known in sophisticated medical jargon as cell wall deficient organisms. Cell wall deficient organisms are highly destructive to the body. These organisms mutate into the cell wall deficient form as an adaptation to the antibiotic attack. Now, this lack of the cell wall has a number of dire consequences. These consequences include a resistance against drugs as well as the capacity to evade immune surveillance. Simply put, as a result of such mutations the antibiotics no longer work. That's because drugs of the tetracycline class interfere with the bacterial cell's production of that outer coating. Yet, like the antibiotics the immune system response is reliant on that outer cell wall. It is the antigens on the bacterial cell coating that are used by this system to recognize it so it can be attacked and destroyed. When the immune system can no longer see those antigens, as happens in cell wall deficient forms, then, the bacteria become inordinately dangerous. There is no means for the immune system to halt or stall their growth.

Antibiotics: challenges and toxicity from the top experts

The problem with medical therapy is one of excesses. Since there is little which is truly effective in medicine for chronic disease, if there is a modestly effective therapy, such as antibiotics, it is extensively overused. This is surely the case with Lyme disease, where antibiotics are used aggressively and often excessively.

Apparently, for Lyme infection victims these drugs even cause significant toxicity to the brain. The degree of toxicity is dependent upon the extensiveness of use. Much of the breakthrough research in this regard has been conducted by a medical clinic specializing in Lyme disease treatment, Florida's Sponaugle Wellness Institute. According to the Institute's website its medical researchers have "analyzed over 8000 brain chemistry patterns" in Lyme disease victims. Through this analysis it has been discovered that Lyme patients have *antibiotic-induced changes in brain chemistry*. These changes result, according to the Institute, in excessive electrical activity in two specific brain regions. Symptoms of such overactivity include depression, anxiety, moodiness, agitation, obsessiveness, a sense of hopelessness, and a tendency to worry excessively. Many of these symptoms are likely a consequence of toxicity to candida yeast toxins.

As a result of infestation of the gut and other tissue linings by candida Lyme patients often end up suffering to a greater degree than if they wouldn't have taken the antibiotics. They became, essentially, a fungal brewery leading to additional production of candidal toxins. The yeast overgrowth results in the suppression of immune function, making it virtually impossible for the body to fight off any remnants of Lyme. In particular, such drug therapy results in a suppression of the natural vigorousness of white blood cells. As a result the body can readily be overcome by virtually any infestation, including the resurgence of mutated and/or antibiotic-resistant tick-borne spirochetes.

Yet, doctors claim the antibiotics cure. Perhaps this is because they create the appearance of therapeutic success. The Lyme can no longer be detected, and the symptoms appear, at least initially, to be suppressed. Even so, clearly, in many cases as a result of multiple courses of antibiotics the disease is far from resolved. As demonstrated by the Sponaugle Wellness Institute the victims of Lyme "often become more debilitated" than they would have been otherwise as a result of "months of aggressive antibiotic therapy." Once again, this is largely a consequence of infestation by candida and other yeasts.

Regardless, it is not possible for the patient to prevail merely with antibiotic therapy with no other supportive care. As a result of the induction of yeast infestation the standard treatment results in great damage to the intestinal canal. How can anyone function adequately with damaged, inflamed, and infested intestines? This is where all the digestion and absorption of nutrients occurs.

Drug therapy leads to the creation of not only mutated candida but also bacterial mutants. All such mutants colonize the gut wall, displacing the healthy bacteria, creating a condition known as dysbiosis.

The dysbiosis is highly damaging. In this regard it should be realized that the gut is not only for digestion but is also a key element of the immune system. Some 60% of the immune organ is located in the intestinal canal, specifically in the lining of the small intestine. This gut-based immune component is known as the Peyer's Patches and consists of a dense concentration of lymphoid tissue.

The Peyer's Patches are the key body organ for the production of the all-important antibodies. They also aid in the production of lymphocytes, which are essential in particular for combating cancer and viral infections.

For the cure of Lyme disease all that is possible must be done to bolster the function of these lymphoid tissue patches, not diminish them. One way they are greatly diminished is through the destruction of the good intestinal bacteria, known as lactobacillus and bifidobacillus.

Yet, what do antibiotics do? They systematically destroy such good bacteria while doing nothing to deal with their ultimate enemies: pathogenic yeasts. Through the production of a variety of toxins these yeasts drive out the healthy bacteria, essentially, permanently. These yeast-produced poisons are known as mycotoxins. The mycotoxins are exceedingly poisonous and are capable of disrupting the function of all organs in the body. These noxious substances are readily destroyed through the intake of edible, food-grade oil of wild oregano.

The lactobacillus produce a compound essential to optimal intestinal health known as lactic acid. It is this acidic substance which is responsible for maintaining the normal pH of the intestines. This is an acidic pH; the acidic environment prevents the overgrowth of pathogens, including yeasts. The yeasts favor an alkaline environment and so, therefore, flourish as a result of the antibiotic treatment. It is a double whammy; the antibiotics kill the good bacteria and halt, as a consequence, all lactic acid production, leading to a vast alteration in normal gut ecology.

In contrast, wild oregano has an acidic reaction. It works with probiotic supplementation to repress the overgrowth of pathogenic yeasts. Too, wild oregano oil can suppress healthy bacterial growth but only in high doses. Plus, with wild oregano oil and other spice oil therapy this repression is reversible.

Certain noxious bacteria also thrive in an alkaline environment. These disease-causing bacteria include clostridium, klebsiella, enterobacteria, and proteus. Like the yeasts such bacteria corrupt the normal environment of the intestinal walls, leading to toxicity and disease.

As the infestation of the aberrant germs becomes extreme, damage occurs to the gut wall. This includes damage and corruption of the intestinal system's immune organ, the Peyer's Patches.

It's a vicious cycle. The antibiotics lead to the infestation of the wrong types of organisms. These organisms damage the gut wall, while overwhelming the local immunity. The immunity of the gut is now fully compromised; it cannot respond to toxicity, assaults, allergens, and noxious germs. The germs then more deeply invade the intestinal membranes. They actually bore holes in such membranes. This leads to a condition known as Leaky Gut Syndrome.

Because of the compromised nature of the highly protective Peyer's Patches, antibody production is diminished. Thus, there are less defenses available to block the further invasion of the intestines by a host of pathogens, including yeasts, viruses, and parasites.

As a result of candida overgrowth the nutrients are poorly absorbed. Despite a potentially healthy diet the individual becomes malnourished. In particular, there develops deficiencies of amino acids, which are essential for the building of immune cells and antibodies.

Why antibiotics fail: the biofilm element

What is a biofilm? It is a microbially-produced film or layer that is virtually impenetrable. It is a protective mechanism used by germs to block any attack by other germs and/or natural immunity. How can germ-killing or -inhibiting drugs work if the germ surrounds itself with a sticky, impenetrable film?

The film is a kind of matrix or matting produced by the germ in which it surrounds itself. Exceedingly sticky, it is made from sugars bound together, known as a polysaccharide matrix. It's a novel production and its existence effectively prevents the immune system from eradicating the germ.

For the germ to be killed the biofilm must be dissolved. This is precisely what the oil of wild oregano achieves, as it is a potent solvent fully capable of dissolving all germ biofilms. Other spices capable of such dissolution include oils of wild sage and bay leaf.

Failure number two: the multiplicity of germs

How can antibiotics work for Lyme when it is caused by a multiplicity of germs, including those never killed by such drugs? Who could possibly believe that as a result of a tick bite only the Lyme spirochete is contracted? With its rodent blood-based infestations, surely a multiplicity of pathogens, known and unknown, are contracted with each tick bite.

In fact, new, novel germ infections resultant from tick bites are being discovered routinely. Consider the cases of mysterious illnesses contracted by Missouri farmers. As reported in 2014 in 2009 two such farmers were known to contract a 'strange' illness manifested by high fever, diarrhea, and nausea, along with a plunge in platelet levels. As in many cases of Lyme antibiotics proved useless for the condition.

Blood was sent to the CDC. When virologists viewed the samples they discovered a virus no one had ever reported before. Further studies confirmed that it was an entity found in the bloodstream and saliva of Missouri ticks, specifically the state's lone star tick. Both farmers had been bitten by ticks before getting sick.

Moreover, it wasn't the adult tick that harbored it. Rather, it was only the tiny nymph which was the source according to an extensive investigation by Harry Savage, M.D., and his team. They studied some 50,000 ticks and confirmed that this, like Lyme, is exclusively a tick bite-based disease.

Near the home of one of the farmers, 1 in 500 nymphs had the virus. "If we were looking for Lyme in Connecticut, there would be more ticks infected," Savage says, "but for a virus [1 in 500], is a substantial number." Savage and his team published their findings in the *American Journal of Tropical Medicine and Hygiene*.

The lone star tick—which is named after the white spot on its back, not Texas—doesn't carry the bacteria that causes Lyme disease. But it has been linked to a similar illness, called Southern tick-associated rash illness. And its bite can leave a rash that looks like the one caused by the Lyme-carrying deer tick.

These toxins are fatty in structure and deposit in the fattiest organ, our brain which is 60 percent fat. These neurotoxins inflame the brain's white matter, the insulation on brain neurons called myelin, adding to the cumulative level of neurotoxicity which is already significant in Lyme patients from brain accumulation of the Lyme toxin. When neurotoxins inflame the myelin sheath of the brain, the electromagnetic field surrounding the neuron is charged, slowing the speed of the electrical impulse. By this mechanism, neurotoxins essentially suppress the brain's electrical activity. In a healthy brain electrical current jumps over the myelin on brain neurons in rapid fashion. However, when the myelin sheath becomes contaminated with neurotoxins from the gut or from toxins of the Lyme spirochete, it fails to effectively modulate immune function. Note: much of this information was gleaned from the write-ups on the website, www.sponauglewellness.com with substantial modifications.

So, antibiotics don't even clear the Lyme germ from the body?

In studies on monkeys it has been determined that antibiotics do not induce a complete cure. In fact, in one investigation where the animals were treated for some 28 days *Borrelia burgdorferi* persisted as an infectious agent in all the monkeys who were treated, in this case with doxycycline. This was in monkeys who were treated after they contracted the diseases some four months after they were infected. Even after being treated for 90 days with intravenous and then oral antibiotics the majority had persistent infection, some 75% of them. This will be covered later in more detail.

Natural remedies to the rescue

It was a choice, whether to take the antibiotics or trust in the natural cures. Choosing the later, an aggressive course was taken. Initially, the following supplements were taken:

- oil of wild oregano (P73 material)
- multiple spice dried essential oil complex consisting of oils of wild oregano and sage, along with remote-source cumin and cinnamon.
- juice of wild oregano
- whole crude wild oregano with *Rhus coriaria*, garlic, and onion (as multiple spice capsules)
- capsules of antiinflammatory enzymes containing bromelain and papain, along with ginger

> Note: the multiple spice oil dessicated formula is based on research conducted at Georgetown University, where a wide range

> of spice oils were tested against stubborn pathogens. In this research only a few spice oils were found to be universal antiseptics, the most potent of these being wild oregano oil, followed by in order of aggressiveness oils of sage, bay leaf, cumin, and cinnamon.

It seemed like a sufficient protocol. Yet, the results were initially minimal at best. The condition seemed to stabilize, which was a positive result. Even so, initially, the Lyme didn't seem to be responding dramatically. It was slow and agonizing. The wild oregano and multiple spice therapy put the horror into a stall. Essentially, it prevented my hospitalization.

Despite this, there was frustration. Wild oregano had always obliterated any other condition previously, doing so precipitously. What was going on, here? The improvement—the normalization—was slow in coming. How could that be?

The ankle was still seized up, the shoulders painful, and now there was involvement of the elbow. Because of the pain and inflammation in the shoulder and elbow it was difficult to dress into a shirt. The slightest degree of stress caused a worsening in the pain. Moreover, the rash, the infernal rash. It burned; it was so uncomfortable. There was no way to sleep in comfort. The nights were a matter of agony. I kept rubbing the wild oregano oil on it, also wild chaga cream. They helped somewhat.

How could it be this bad? How could any such disease be this difficult?

The head still did not feel right. It seemed obvious that the spirochete was infecting the brain tissue as well as the spinal cord. For this the wild oregano oil was taken sublingually repeatedly, along with the multiple spice dried oil capsules. Finally, the head and spinal pain began to ease, thanks to the power of these natural medicines.

A high quality calcium bentonite clay poultice was applied on my mid-thoracic spine as a new battle plan. This had a strong drawing action and aided in easing the spinal and cranial pain (available exclusively from powerhourmall.com). It began to become clear that the disease would not achieve its seemingly murderous aim. With the increasing of the dose of the multiple spice complex and the addition of the clay poultice improvement was slow, but it was steady and significant.

Because of the nature of the Lyme spirochete, along with the existence of numerous co-infections, this disease is truly a challenge. There is also the issue of the suspected weaponized nature of the germ, where its infectivity is seemingly greatly enhanced as well as its ability to evade immune defenses. This is why, clearly, Lyme poses a far greater challenge in terms of cure and eradication versus other bacterial infections. Now, it is clear from later experimentation that the addition of the whole, crude wild oregano with *Rhus coriaria* speeds up the rate of cure.

All this exemplifies the challenges facing Lyme disease victims. High invasiveness, weaponization, immune evasion, a high degree of penetrating capacity into the deepest of all tissues, high destructive capacity against the tissues and organs: no wonder the suffering and agony is so great.

So, when the constellation of symptoms strike, so seemingly deadly—so resistant to every conceivable therapeutic approach—what is a person to do? No wonder people submit to month upon month of antibiotic therapy in hope for a miracle cure. Here, in this book there is no attempt to dissuade people from such therapy. It is merely the point that doctors don't know what else to do for patients, and, here, other options are provided.

The propensity of the bacteria for the spinal tissue and fluids is one of its most ominous aspects. Equally dire, though, is the proclivity of the bacillus for the brain tissue. Victims of Lyme must constantly deal with the consequence of this infectivity, that is unless full eradication can be achieved. The bacteria may reside chronically in such tissues and use these tissues as the launching site to continuously infect the body. It is not easy for the body to root out such germs trapped in the spinal tissues, spinal fluid, and brain tissue. This requires a major effort, with a reliance on natural cures that can help the body systematically root out such infestation. Yet, this rooting out must be achieved. Otherwise, the individual will suffer forever with the infection. In the event of such infestation one substance to add to the protocol is the juice of wild oregano. This aromatic essence has the capacity to penetrate the blood brain barrier.

The human body has no innate immunity against the Lyme spirochete. That is because it is a biologically altered germ. This demonstrates the need for use of every conceivable therapy known, whether orthodox or alternative

To prevail against the Lyme biogerm every conceivable power must be leveraged. In this regard wild oregano oil, edible type, high mountain-Mediterranean-source, is ideal, along with wild turmeric extract, and various multiple spice formulas, along with the whole, crude herb plus *Rhus coriaria* as 600 mg capsules. For the maximum benefits all must be utilized: even alongside antibiotics. Other wild medicines which may prove invaluable in the reversal of this disease include wild cat's claw powder (12:1 concentrate), wild chaga, wild larch bark, black seed oil, wild far northern Canadian hyssop, wild teasel root, wild yarrow, and wild, raw freshwater cod liver oil as a whole liver extract.

Cat's claw itself is an antiseptic, being derived from bark. Thus, it is an ideal addition to the wild spice oil therapy.

The appropriate, nutrient-rich diet is also necessary in reversing the disease. Since Lyme leads to a breakdown in tissues, including their degeneration, the diet must be aimed at inducing organ regeneration. There is need for the richest of all foods, those with dense supplies of nutrients: the B complex, minerals, vitamins A and D, vitamin C, fatty acids, amino acids, and more. Such a diet is known as a nutrient dense diet. Necessarily, this type of diet includes animal-source foods, although such foods must arise exclusively from entirely natural sources. In contrast, a vegan diet is low in nutrient density and is not the preferable type in the battle to conquer this disease.

For the regeneration of damaged tissue, as well as the activation and strengthening of the immune system, the essential amino acids found in milk products are of value. In most cases it is not milk itself that is needed, especially in the case of lactose intolerance, but rather, in particular, fermented milk products such as yogurt, kefir, and quark. These milk products must arise exclusively from entirely natural and/or organic sources. In general those from goat's and sheep's milk are more readily tolerated than cow's milk sources. In fact, any foods rich in the healthy bacteria, that is lactobacillus species—sauerkraut, for instance—are of great importance in creating the necessary intestinal environment to achieve the cure.

Even so, milk products are not for everyone. Some people are highly sensitive to milk protein, others lactose intolerant. Also, the Lyme bacillus has been found in diseased cows. It may cross contaminate into the milk. If cow's milk products are consumed, they should be from healthy, organically raised herds. For those who are sensitive to milk products other options include the consumption of organic sources of red meat and poultry. It is best to individualize any program, and foods that are tolerated must be the focus. In the event of milk allergy plant proteins may be the best option such as sprouted brown rice powder, pea protein, or others. Yet, for those who can tolerate it milk protein is an ideal source of all eight essential amino acids needed for tissue repair and is more efficiently used for such repair than vegetable sources.

Vegetable sources of protein, such as hemp and brown rice protein powders, are also important. However, they are devoid of the full spectrum of sulfur-bearing amino acids found in rich supplies in the protein of meat, poultry, eggs, and milk. Such amino acids, for instance, cysteine, are essential for the repair of damaged muscles and joints. Adding a raw egg to a brown rice-hemp protein drink would make it more complete.

The protein from eggs can be invaluable as a rebuilding agent. In this case only organically raised eggs must be used. The whole raw egg can be added to a protein shake. Here is a raw egg drink that can be consumed regularly for purposes of regeneration. It is a rich and delicious drink and may be used as a sole meal, for instance, as a breakfast:

2 raw organic eggs, either whole or the yolks only
cup organic yogurt
1 T. Purely-B natural B complex powder
1 T. sprouted brown rice-hemp protein powder
1 T. raw honey or one or two tsp. raw yacon syrup
frozen or fresh berries

In a blender blend until smooth. Drink as a whole meal or as an adjunct to breakfast. Or, use as a between-meals power and energy booster.

Are all tick bites potentially lethal?

Countless people have suffered bites by non-Lyme infested ticks. Most such people endured these bites without the slightest incident or in some cases modest symptoms such as localized inflammation and swelling. With such a proclivity for hunting in the wilderness there were numerous times where I have contracted tick-related conditions. In all cases the tick was discovered, killed, and removed. Years prior to this latest event in one case the removal was left to a worker. He pulled it out inappropriately, leaving the head remaining. A Lyme-like syndrome developed, which manifested not with the standard symptoms but, rather those related to the heart. Severe cardiac pain, actual angina, developed. This could have represented invasion of the spirochete into the heart muscle itself, a condition known as cardiac Lyme. Yet, it was quickly obliterated through a course of spice oil therapy, including the vigorous consumption of wild juice of oregano, about a half bottle per day for a week, plus a hefty dosage of the super-strength form of the oil as drops under the tongue. The oil dosage was 40 drops several times daily. In particular, regarding this condition the juice has a power which is novel; it increases the muscular pumping power of the heart. For the heart muscle pump and the circulation, additionally, red sour grape powder was taken as capsules, 4 capsules three times daily. Also, the mountain-grown Mediterranean pomegranate molasses was consumed, about four tablespoons daily.

The results were at first gradual but highly noticeable. The angina began to quickly dissipate. The 'cardiac fear' began to wane. Within a month I was back to normal.

In another case a wood tick attacked the posterior aspect of my ear near the mastoid process. Even though it was properly removed, actually, it was killed with a super-strength form of oil of wild oregano by saturating that oil on a cotton ball and holding it against the tick until it died, then removing it. Even so, two days later I fell ill. In this case the entire left side of my body went paralyzed. It was physically impossible to move that left side; a kind of Guillain Barré syndrome had developed, very frightening.

It made sense. The tick had lodged itself on the temporal bone area near the ear cartilage on the right side. Right-sided infection will travel through the circulation to the left brain. Also, tick spirochetes and other pathogens have the capacity of traveling through the nerve sheaths. Infections on the right side of the body will cause left-sided neurological diseases.

Regardless, when infections from ticks strike, the symptoms arise by surprise. Often, such a presentation begins with neurological symptoms. Suddenly, the person develops numbness on one side of the body. More extremely, there is one-sided paralysis, usually involving both the arm and leg. There may be complete inability to move the leg. "I am paralyzed; my body won't responde to command. This is horrifying," the person will think. "Will I ever be able to walk again?"

The answer is, "Yes." In my case I could not move either the arm or the leg. Thus, an aggressive spice oil therapy was instituted, the exact protocol, as follows:

- juice of wild oregano: two ounces twice daily, although in the first day after the paralysis an entire bottle was consumed (12-ounces)
- juice of wild rosemary: two ounces twice daily
- oil of wild oregano (a super-strength form): two to three droppersful under the tongue several times daily
- antiinflammatory enzymes consisting of bromelain, papain, and others: on an empty stomach three or more capsules three times daily

In every case in the past there was this realization; "Go to old faithful, the wild oregano oil and the aromatic essence, that is steam-extracted juice. This will be sufficient to reverse the tick-infestation syndrome." Moreover, it was always precisely the case that it reliably achieved the results as expected. Too, it did so rapidly, and there was no doubt about the result.

This time it was different. The pathogen(s) was/were more resistant than the others. The Wisconsin case of Lyme took much longer than expected to eradicate. Plus, increasingly massive doses were required in order to merely keep the germ infestation at bay, let alone eradicate it. Thus, it was likely that I was suffering not only with Lyme but also with co-infection syndrome, like bartonella and mycoplasma.

It was different, too, because it was a full-blown case of neuroborreliosis, meaning the spirochete had fully infested the central nervous system. The good news was it was gradually responding. The ankle was no longer stiff. The bull's eye rash had finally gone. It had popped up again in the form of a kind of spotted rash on the chest and torso. However, an increase in the dose of the multiple spice concentrate/extract obliterated it. The fullness of the head and spine was still there but had diminished about 50%. Sleeping was still difficult, with plenty of tossing and turning and a goodly amount of moaning. The moaning seemed to aid the ability to fall asleep. There was some fatigue. The sensation of burning all over the body had diminished greatly but was still there to a lesser degree.

Even after a month of the natural therapy a variety of bizarre sensations persisted. The ability to function and, in particular, to mentally concentrate was disrupted. The joint sequela was now concentrated in the shoulders and elbows. It was difficult to put a shirt on; there was still much weakness and pain in the shoulders and elbows. Too, the elbow became swollen with a Popeye-like presentation. That pocket of swelling drooped down from the elbow joint a full two inches. Finally, in desperation a more radical action was taken.

I drank *an entire bottle*, one ounce, of super-strength oregano oil mixed in water/juice daily for four days. Simultaneously, I took 45 capsules of multiple spice extract daily in divided doses, a half a large bottle daily. In addition, the juice of oregano was vigorously consumed, about three ounces or more per day. Added to this was a healthy bacterial supplement, that is Ecologic 500, two teaspoonsful at night. I also cranked-up the dosage of antiinflammatory enzymes. Finally, after two days of this therapy a dramatic, positive result was seen. It was clear that I was out of the danger zone. The fullness of the head and spinal column were cleared. The stiffness of the deltoids had improved. The swelling in the elbow and the aching in that joint had largely dissipated. I was sleeping better, which was a good sign.

The persistent fatigue and inability to function were now gone. The burning sensation throughout the body was purged, never again to return. Therefore, through the natural wild spice therapy the major manifestations of the disease were conquered. It was as if that immense dosage of wild oregano oil had broken the resistance of the Lyme, saving my life.

Yet, was the Lyme itself in general fully eradicated? In fact, it was not, since the spirochete is capable of surviving in a mutated, encysted form. The symptoms were now seemingly limited to the joint capsules, especially that of the right elbow and shoulder region; in other words, there were still residual issues. Inflammation and pain in these regions, along with swelling of the elbow, were the only remaining symptoms, that is from the original ones associated with the affliction. Even so, at this point there was a 70% improvement, which was highly encouraging.

Despite this, it was some two months after the mega-dose therapy that the elbow swelling recurred. In this case it was the size of a small orange. It seemed to represent a kind of attempt by the Lyme to resurface. Actually, it was a sign that it was still hidden in the body, operating to cause corruption through stealth.

Deep in the joint there was great pain and discomfort to pressure. The swelling area was not painful. Still, the mobility of the entire right shoulder and elbow area was slightly diminished. There was, though, only a modest amount of pain upon movement. In fact, there seemed to be virtually fully normal movement in the elbow and shoulder. It was just that there was a deep ache and a kind of weakness. It was a weakness noticeable especially when grabbing an item, as if it would slip from the hand. This was likely a consequence of the spirochete's attack on the nerve centers.

After a month there was a relapse in one of the symptoms. It was the swelling of the elbow. The swelling was hideous. absolutely pathological. The underside of the elbow joint was just one blob of puffiness. Thus, once again, aggressive action was taken. People said, "Go to the doctor and get that tapped." Just tap the fluid? How will that cure infection and inflammation? How will sticking a needle into a single joint solve a condition which is systemic, which affects to some degree every tissue and organ of the body?

Thus, a different approach was taken, which is primarily through oral dosing. Increasingly massive doses of the multiple spice capsules, once again, 30 to 45 capsules daily with food and/or juice sometimes also on an empty stomach were consumed. Note: for those with sensitive stomachs do take this with juice and or food. Within a week of this therapy the swelling was completely eliminated. Even so, the weakness upon grabbing an item—the inability, to hold a heavy item tightly—persisted.

Additionally, though there was no obvious pain in the swollen blob there was pain upon deep pressure. This was elicited by pressure on the radial head and also about the ulnar bone on the underside of the elbow.

Those were the obvious symptoms. Despite the dramatic improvements it was realized that there still could be the spirochete hiding within the brain and spinal cord. That could explain the weakness of both shoulders and the inability to hold onto objects. It could also explain the tendency to relapse upon stress.

When bumping into an object on the right side of the arm at the elbow joint, there was extreme pain. Incredibly, the mind was strong, and there was the desire to do more with the body in terms of moving, lifting, and even exercising. Yet, the body did not cooperate with the mind-power. All such symptoms are typical of infestation of the nervous system by the Lyme spirochete. These are also the kinds of symptoms seen in multiple sclerosis and, particularly, Lou Gehrig's disease (ALS). Even so, clearly, I was now 80% better, that is versus where I started, and was in nowhere near the kind of danger zone that had developed during the initial course of the disease.

It seemed that the right shoulder girdle had been somehow injured by the Lyme. In speaking with other victims this is apparently not uncommon. Several Lyme sufferers reported that they had lost significant shoulder function, which included the loss of muscle tissue, known as muscular atrophy.

The question was how to eliminate the symptoms while inducing healing in the shoulder joint system. Or, was this more dire than it seemed? Was the spirochete still lodged in the central nervous system, infecting and irritating the shoulder capsule through axoplasmic flow?

The previous but now eradicated swelling of the elbow was indicative of actual tissue damage in the joint, the fluid being produced as a kind of consequence of such damage. That eradication was achieved incredibly without antibiotics and was exclusively due to the massive intake of the multiple spice extract, along with the super-strength oil of oregano, the juice of wild oregano, and various other supportive supplements, including the oil of wild turmeric. Additionally, the oil of oregano in an extra virgin olive oil base was vigorously rubbed on the elbow and shoulder joints repeatedly, as was the deep-eezing multiple spice rubbing oil. Also, about 40 drops in the palm of such an oil complex was held against the elbow joint in the areas of the greatest pain and soreness. This greatly aided the healing process, although the internal intake proved to be most effective in achieving overall eradication.

More recently, another wild herbal medicine has become in vogue. Known as wild teasel root, this powerful medicine is a definite aid in the reversal of Lyme. Available as a two ounce tincture, ideally, seek a teasel root supplement that is extracted with natural substances, such as virgin olive oil and cider vinegar, versus those extracted with alcohol and glycerin.

Clearly, tick bites are a great and unprecedented danger to the people of this world. In many instances it is such an incredibly difficult struggle to overcome tick-induced diseases. This demonstrates the value of prevention, that is not getting bit.

Chapter Seven

Preventive Medicine

When considering prevention it is worth reiterating the devastating nature of this condition and how it attacks multiple systems of the body. The work of medical author William C. Shiel, who published the article, along with editor M. C. Stoppler, *Lyme Disease*, is demonstrative in this regard. In their review they make it clear that, firstly, while the condition is mainly caused by the Lyme bacteria it may also involve, as is well published, numerous co-infections. The major destruction is inflicted upon the "skin, *joints*, heart, and *nervous system*." Then, too, Shiel notes, importantly, the disease occurs in stages or phases, the earliest one being at the actual site of the tick bite. At this site in many cases there develops "an expanding ring of redness." This is where the initial infestation occurs.

This area should ideally be treated to minimize the spread of disease, in this case with the oil of wild oregano (super-strength) and also by taking the oil internally, along with the juice of oregano and the multiple spice dessicated oil complex.

Any tick bite region, if discovered, should be treated topically. The tick itself, along with the bite area, should be saturated with the oil of wild oregano to attain constant contact, which is ideal to destroy any residual tick-related germs and the consequential local inflammation. That constant contact can also be achieved by saturating a bandage or a piece of cotton and once the tick is removed taping the saturated cotton against the region. This can then be changed every 12 or 24 hours and continued until all infection and inflammation is eradicated.

In my case the infection was realized too late, that is for a quick and easy cure to be affected. If there had been a realization that there was a tick bite plus infestation immediately, all the consequences could have been avoided. Therefore, I suffered needlessly for over a year with various symptoms, all because the bite and the resultant infection were in operation through stealth.

The point is that because of the danger of this disease extraordinary efforts must be made to protect against the consequences. No effort or method should be spared that has the potential to prevent tick bites.

Natural cures are a positive option, not a danger

I was once at a sale, in fact, an estate liquidation when a liquidator, a friend of mine, noticed that I was not my old self. This was at a point where the Lyme condition was only about 40% reversed. Purchasing some garden decorations made of heavy material, I mentioned to the estate agent that I had Lyme and that lifting posed a real challenge. She offered a young man as a helper.

Meanwhile, a woman who overheard this looked at me with a degree of shock in her eyes. “Don’t worry, I’m treating it naturally with herbal medicines, oil of wild oregano and more.”

"You mean you're not taking antibiotics?," she quipped. "Do you have any idea what your are saying? You are playing with fire; Lyme is deadly," at which point, once again, she gave me an astonished look, this time almost of disgust.

"It will be alright," I responded. "The natural cures, God-given herbs, will reverse it. I'll be fine," at which point the woman turned around and walked away.

Now, it is true that Lyme is a devastating disease, which can prove fatal. Yet, too, it is often chronic and insidious. This is why the use of natural remedies is ideal. What other options do people have who choose not to take prolonged courses of potentially noxious antibiotics?

Prevention: the key

For thousands of years humanity has enjoyed wilderness environments, in many cases without the slightest risk of danger. The exception might be tropical environments, where mosquito-borne diseases are common, some of which are deadly. Yet, local inhabitants of such forests often develop a kind of immunity to such diseases. It is primarily unaccustomed visitors who readily contract the conditions, malaria, West Nile, and Chaga's disease, for instance. Yet, in the Western world and, in particular, the Northern Hemisphere there were previously essentially no such deadly diseases associated with biting insects, the exception being Rocky Mountain Spotted Fever and a few rare others.

Because of the danger of Lyme and other tick-borne infections, as well as West Nile, it is not possible to fully and freely enjoy the environment in many regions, and this is true of both North America and Europe. The Lyme tick has fully infested vast tracts of these continents. A mere single tick attachment can result in the onset of horrendous disease, which could prove fatal.

That danger is a time-sensitive one. In early spring there is virtually no such danger, as is also true of the late fall. Of course, during winter there is no danger of tick bites. This applies only to areas in the Northern Hemisphere. In more temperate regions the danger of tick bites may exist continuously.

In the Northern Hemisphere what are the months of the greatest risk? They are May, June, and July. There is also a significant risk for deer tick bites, and bites by wood ticks, in August, that risk declining dramatically by mid-September. In some areas even early spring, such as mid-April, poses a risk.

This is a serious issue. Therefore, people must now deliberate over taking any excursion into the wilderness. Precautions must be taken. The appropriate routines must be followed. It is no longer safe to in a nonchalant manner go out into the woods and, for instance, have a "picnic." It is all thanks to the criminal minds associated with Plum Island.

Precautions and protections

There are a number of steps that can be taken to achieve protection against tick and mosquito bites. These protective steps are as follows:

Ticks

- Wear the lightest-colored clothes possible, preferably white or off-white. White is the best, since the tiny tick nymphs, which are black, can be seen more readily. Larger ticks can be easily seen against such a background.
- Always take the time to do the specialized sock-protection routine. Here, the socks are pulled over the pant legs. The

socks should be white.

- Spray the shoes, socks, and legs with the natural, potent tick repellent, Herbal Tick-X. This combination of essential and spice oils truly is effective in repelling ticks, especially the highly infective nymph.
- Check clothes often for evidence of crawling, climbing ticks.
- Wear a hat to prevent ticks from falling from tall grass or trees onto the head.
- Be sensitive, and be aware. Have a high awareness for entities crawling on the body or in the hair. If any such sensations occur, check the body immediately.
- Upon arriving home or when in a secure place, strip down immediately; place all clothing in a plastic bag. Inspect the body fully for ticks. Too, the head and neck should be carefully inspected. The hair should be thoroughly brushed and/or combed all the way down to the scalp. After any wilderness adventure take a shower and scrub the skin and hair vigorously.

Mosquitoes

- Avoid the consumption of refined sugar prior to the wilderness excursion. Such sugar creates the environment in the blood, a sweetness, favoring mosquito attacks.
- Do not eat bananas. This fruit contains aromatic compounds which attract mosquitoes.
- Eat foods rich in B complex, notably brown rice, organic liver, organic or free range eggs, cheese, and yeast.
- Take a whole food B complex powder such as Purely B, two or more tablespoonsful daily; the B vitamin thiamine in particular is an antagonist to mosquito attack.

- Use goodly amounts of spices in foods, including oregano, thyme, basil, turmeric, clove, cinnamon, and more; mosquitoes are repelled by the scent of spices.
- Protect the exposed parts of the body with clothing as much as possible. Wear a type of clothing that prevents the insect from biting through; protect the back especially.
- Burn aromatic devices, such as those which are citronella-based, if camping or in a stationary area.
- Make aggressive use of a spice oil-based mosquito repellent, particularly Herbal Tick-X. This is a highly effective formula that is often just as effective, if not more effective, than the petrochemical-based types especially against mosquitoes. If you must use DEET, use the two together to reduce the amount of the petrochemical derivative applied. This spice oil formula is entirely safe and can even be applied to babies and infants. Furthermore, it may be applied repeatedly, as often as needed.

Additionally, be sure to have available a bottle of super-strength potency oil of wild oregano and/or the liquid multiple spice formula consisting of oils of wild oregano and sage, along with cinnamon and cumin. If a tick is attached, saturate a piece of cotton, gauze, or paper towel, then apply it to the tick. Hold it there continuously until the insect dies.

It takes some 10 to 20 minutes of contact to kill the tick. This is an extremely valuable method; it greatly reduces the risk of the spread of infection from the typical way of dealing with an attached tick, which is handling it while it is alive and still attached. Even so, if it is barely attached, it could be removed immediately without the spice oil treatment. If it is deeply attached, handling it may lead to the additional injection of tick secretions, as the insect struggles and wiggles against contact. Too, it is not easy to remove a live tick that is well embedded into the tissues without increasing the risks for such a spread. A dead tick is readily extracted, simply with the tweezers applied firmly to the body. A gentle pulling removes the tick and all its parts.

Alternatively, the tick can be saturated with the natural antiseptic spray, Germ-a-Clenz, which will also kill it. Essentially, the contact with the hot spice oil complex—or the wild oregano oil—suffocates the tick to death.

Despite all these precautions it is still possible to get Lyme disease, even though the odds will be reduced significantly. One aid in powerful prevention would be to take the oil of wild oregano prophylactically during tick season, as in drops under the tongue or edible gelcaps (60 mg of total extra virgin olive oil and oregano oil per capsule). Another protection would be the intake of the multiple spice capsules containing oils of wild oregano and sage plus cumin and cinnamon.

In this regard it is worth reviewing one of the key signs, one which is absolutely definitive. This is the bull's eye rash. If the rash is shaped like a bull's eye, whether circular or oval with the edge being darkest at the outside margin, this is 100% definitive proof of Lyme. The challenge is that this definitive rash is only seen in some 40% of instances.

This rash starts usually a few days after the tick attachment. Yet, it could develop much later, up to several weeks afterwards. In oval or circular rings the rash often expands over several days, becoming several inches long. The concentric rings represents the typical appearance. In some cases it takes on a bruise-like appearance. Furthermore, the Lyme rash may be confused with spider bites as well as cellulitis.

In some cases the rash may appear in multiple regions, so-called satellite rashes. There are even cases where there is initially the large rash followed by such satellite lesions. Even so, the development of the rash means that a serious Lyme infection is developing.

Another virtually definitive sign of the condition is the sudden, unexplained onset of Bell's palsy. This represents a toxicity and/or infection by this germ of the cranial nerve known as the facial nerve. Yet another is a flu-like syndrome associated with joint pain occurring in the early- to mid-summer.

The chronic symptoms are more vague and could readily be represented by other conditions. These symptoms include stiff neck, headache, joint stiffness, joint pain, swelling of joints, sensitivity to sound or light, impairment of mental function, including a cloudy-like sensation in the brain, poor concentration, bizarre disturbances in sleep, anxiety (which can be extreme), depression, tingling, burning/shooting pains, the sudden onset of generalized arthritis, stiffness of the spine, abdominal pain, nausea, and diarrhea. There may also be symptoms relative to the cardiac and lung systems, including shortness of breath, palpitations, and chest pain. No wonder the condition is frequently misdiagnosed as a wide range of other syndromes. In this regard it surely must be held as a great falsifier, that is a condition which mimics more conditions than can be named (for a complete list of Lyme disease symptoms see Appendix A).

Chapter Eight

Is Lyme Weaponized Syphilis?

It has been established, here, that, like syphilis, Lyme mimics a vast number of diseases. This is a result of the insidious nature of the infection, as the Lyme spirochete alters its state, morphologically, to cause a state of chronic infection and inflammation. The immune system being thus destabilized, virtually any syndrome could develop, which would cause great confusion in diagnosis.Through personal experience with the disease it easy to recognize at least some of the diseases it mimics. These diseases include chronic fatigue syndrome, fibromyalgia, tendonitis, synovitis, single joint arthritis, rheumatoid arthritis, Guillain-Barré syndrome, ALS, polymyalgia rheumatica, and MS. This writer experienced a degree of all of these. Too, just as syphilis methodically eats away at the body, so does Lyme. In fact, syphilis does cause the same kind of presentation as seen in Lyme, particularly neuroborreliosis.

In 1913 Noguchi demonstrated the presence of *Treponema pallidum* (syphilitic spirochete) in the brain of a progressive paralysis patient, proving that the spirochete was the cause of the disease.

A number of other investigators have determined its disease mimics, including the M.D.s Jo Anne Whitaker and Svetlana Ivanova. Their compiled list of potential Lyme disease- and/or co-infection infestation-induced conditions and/or syndromes includes:

acrodermatitis chronica atrophicans (ACA)
Alzheimer's disease
Bell's palsy
irritable bowel syndrome
lupus
Parkinson's disease
reflex sympathetic dystrophy
scleroderma
syphilis
acute atrioventricular block
arrhythmia
attention deficit disorder
attention deficit hyperactivity disorder
Tourette's syndrome
cranial polyneuritis
chronic depression
anxiety neurosis
encephalopathy
insomnia and other sleeping disorders
visual deterioration
meningitis
myocarditis
cardiomyopathy
neuritis

That is a massive number of conditions, and there surely are others besides those which Lyme infection mimics. Yet, this list alone proves the great corruption caused by this pathogen, giving even greater cause for the value of spice oils as preventive and therapeutic agents.

The joint pathology is also variable. Often, it begins in the knee. In fact, swelling in the knee, along with pain and stiffness combined with fatigue, is virtually confirmatory of the disease. At any point, though, it might strike new joint areas. This is true both of early and late presentations. Other joints which are commonly attacked by the Lyme bacillus include the hips, elbows, ankles, wrists, spinal column, and TMJ. Weight-bearing joints are typically compromised. People can be readily crippled by the disease, even ending up wheelchair-bound. This is particularly true when the Lyme bacillus attacks the knee joints.

From the aforementioned it becomes clear that the three systems hit hardest in Lyme disease are the joints, the skin, and the nervous system but also the immune system, which is severely battered by the spirochete. It is also important to note that the attack on the joints can come in bouts. A week or even weeks after the tick bite, suddenly, without any trauma or other obvious cause a joint or several joints become swollen, painful, and inflamed. It truly is a disease by stealth.

The swelling and pain caused by the Lyme invader are bizarre. An involved joint can become dramatically swollen, causing a great degree of pain. Parts around the joint are exceedingly painful to touch. In the knee the aching from the swelling can become intense, brutally so. Other than in that highly destructive disease rheumatoid arthritis it is a novel kind of pain, swelling, and inflammation not seen in any other syndrome. The pain it seems, arises from the deepest recesses of the joint sockets; clearly, the Lyme spirochete is clearly deeply invading the joint capsule, where it hides. In fact, the germ seems to have a predilection for human connective tissue. There is some evidence that it consumes it as food. As a result of such a diabolical attack the capsule tissues respond with the production of excessive amounts of synovial fluid. This fluid accumulates in the joint capsule, leading to swelling and pain.

The only way to fully cure such joint corruption is to completely clear the Lyme spirochete from the body. People often don't know what they are dealing with. Most doctors don't know that the vague joint symptomology and pathology could be borrelia. Lyme is essentially syphilis-like infection, the former also being caused by a spirochete, known medically as *Treponema pallidum*. Lyme was created on the basis of the spirochete as a novel pathogen. It is seemingly a form of syphilis. Like the latter, it can be transmitted sexually. Too, just as there is a condition in syphilis known as neuro-syphilis, that is infestation of the brain and spinal cord with the syphilitic spirochete, the same occurs in Lyme, that is neuroborreliosis. Plus, it is a chronic kind of infestation, meaning that the brain and spinal cord are under continuous siege by the pathogen, which preferentially multiplies in such tissues.

A war must be waged to root such spirochetes out of the nervous system tissue. These germs are geared for readily invading nerve cells. This may explain the fact that Lyme frequently relapses as a result of stress, since the latter weakens the immune capacities of such cells as well as the cells of the bone marrow and immune system itself.

It is crucial to root it out, but it is also essential to strengthen the cells of the brain, spinal cord, and peripheral nerves. Too, it is crucial to strengthen the blood-brain barrier. This can be done through the proper diet along with nutritional supplementation, the supplements being derived exclusively from whole food sources and/or super-foods. Lyme spirochete has a significant capacity to breech this barrier. That's why it is essential to empower it, to strengthen it to the maximum degree.

That breeching occurs in far more cases than is recognized. In fact, according to the latest research it is not merely neuro-Lyme that is caused by borrelia organism but, rather, entire categories of neuroglical diseases as well—Bell's palsy, MS, ALS, and more.

The borrelia genus has been a subject of biowarfare experimentation at least as far back as WW2, when the infamous Japanese Unit 731, which studied its effects experimented on live prisoners. It has already been mentioned that the CDC declared the species a bioweapon, that is "a potential bioterrorism agent."

When the original posting (page 39) was pointed out to the CDC by astute investigators, what was its response? It scrubbed the information from the Internet, claiming it was a mistake. This would appear to be hard proof of a conspiracy of silence, in fact, cover-up.

It must be no surprise that such powerful ones would behave this way. Consider the history of the so-called U.S. Government in regard to the experimentation on the population with biologically altered germs. It's corrupt, make no mistake about it. In a thorough assessment by James Howenstine crucial evidence for this was revealed. The fact is a nation which is developing biologic warfare agents can't just do so in a bubble. The agents must be tested, not merely on animals but also on humans themselves. If the agent could be proven to be effective in corrupting human health and in particular if it can be proven to be transmissible from human to human, then it would be deemed a monumental success.

Noted Howenstine, in WWII in the Faroe Islands British biowarfare researchers ran tests to see if sheep could be infected by air-borne brucella. The sheep did contract it, but then it spread into the sheep dogs, and from there it spread to humans. Several cases of human multiple sclerosis were then tied to the biogerm test. It is reminiscent of Lyme and how neurological conditions have broken out to a pandemic degree since the launching of biowarfare tests on Plum Island.

After the war, about 1947 through 1948, some 1100 teenage school children in remote northern Icelandic villages (Akureyri) became violently ill with a *new disease* manifested by severe burning pain in the limbs, profound muscle weakness, and severe fatigue. Of these, five developed an aggressive form of Parkinson's disease, ultimately dying, which was unheard of in healthy teenagers on the island. At the time the United States had effective control of Iceland. There, a research scientist trained in plant and animal virology at the Rockefeller Institute, Dr. Bjorn Sigurdson, was installed to start an Institute of Experimental Pathology at the University of Iceland. Given a $200,000 grant from the Rockefeller Institute he was purportedly to study different germs on farm animals in the attempt to create, ostensibly, antidotes. Clearly, then, it was the Rockefeller-sponsored research that was the cause of this deadly outbreak.

In the 1950s the Canadian government established in Ontario the Dominion Parasite Laboratory. The purpose was, incredibly, to grow tens of millions of mosquitos each month. The mosquitos were apparently being studied as potential bioweapons. In August 1984 some 500 persons in the St. Lawrence Valley became ill with a mystery illness. Symptoms included extreme weakness, the kind seen in biowarfare disease brucellosis, but no evidence of brucella infection could be found. One victim insisted that her illness resulted from a mosquito bite. She recalled being bitten by a mosquito, waking up the next day with a target skin lesion at the bite site, the same type of lesion as seen in Lyme. She developed such profound weakness she was unable to get out of bed. Still another woman confirmed a target lesion at the mosquito bite site. Neither of the women recovered from their devastating conditions. Clearly, they were sicked by the mosquitos which were turned into biowarfare agents.

Chronic fatigue: a biogerm disease

It gets worse. As pointed out by Howenstine an entire modern epidemic has its origins in biowarfare experimentation. In 1956 citizens in Punta Gorda, Florida, awoke to a horrific nightmare: clouds of mosquitos floating about in their town. Now, here is the incredible part. Calls to the Meteorological Service about the mosquito plague were answered with the information that there had been a forest fire thirty miles away in the Everglades; these mosquitos had fled the fire, it was claimed. Mosquitos never do that. Their range is minimal, forest fires or not. Within a few days five local residents appeared in the media reporting their circumstances, the development of extreme exhaustion, explanation unknown. This was the origin of chronic fatigue syndrome, which was absolutely the result of a biogerm experiment on humans.

Clearly, therefore, the criminals in charge of the powerful elements of the US government do, in fact, perform dangerous experiments upon the American people. The same is true of such hostile elements in Canada. The origin of Lyme is no different. It is the consequence of the unhindered, and unprosecuted, activity of criminal minds.

This brings us to Lyme. It could very well be a consequence of the same kind of corruption. Chronic fatigue syndrome is entirely man-made. Why not Lyme?

Carroll in his book *Lab 257: The Disturbing Story of the Government's Secret Plum Island Germ Laboratory* has provided compelling evidence for just such a corruption. He confirms that the outbreak in the regions near Plum Island could simply not be a coincidence. For the entirety of the 20th century children in Lyme as well as Old Lyme, Connecticut, were free of any such disease. Then, in 1975 in the midst of aggressive vector biowarfare research: then, it breaks out a mere 10 miles away from the lab. That taxpayer-funded building of filthy corruption is the cause of this brutal, murderous pandemic. It is also confirmed by the fact that the outbreak zone is precisely downwind of the lab and its smoke stacks.

In some respects it is astonishing that this didn't happen sooner. Since 1948 ticks were specifically bred, after which they were infected with a wide range of pathogenic agents, including spirochetes. It has always been government-owned, although this might have served as a cover for more nefarious elements such as that terminally corrupt cabal, the Rockefeller family.

From ticks and/or airborne germs of Plum Island in principle there could only be one logical outbreak zone, and that is the area in the direct path of the prevailing oceanic winds which cross the island. That brings us to the shores of Connecticut, in other words, Lyme and Old Lyme.

Carroll demonstrates that at least two provable outbreaks from the lab have reached the mainland, causing corruption of both human and animal life. The outbreak of Lyme has never been admitted or confirmed by 'government' officials. The medical-legal consequences against the lab and its operators would be vast. Too, it is assured that the West Nile virus outbreak originated at the Plum Island facility, and this fact has been routinely disguised.

The epicenter of the pandemic remains in that area, as are the most severe cases which are contracted. Carroll's book is a must read for anyone living in that pandemic zone, and that means all of those living on Long Island, the residents of the eastern half of New York State, and all the residents of Connecticut, New Jersey, and Massachusetts. All such people must take the necessary precautions. As one local has said to me, a New Jersey resident, "Lyme is horrific here, bad beyond belief. People are getting sick from it in huge numbers." Thus, the residents of these states most realize the danger. They must know that when they are anywhere near nature they could be attacked, not by a mere insect, tick, or mosquito but by any biting agent produced for the purposes of harming and killing: a man-made bioweapon.

From work posted by New York State veterinarian Patricia Doyle (Rense.com) there is the following potential confirmation:

> ...Plum Island's work with the "Lone Star Tick," native to Texas. The focal point of experimentation on Plum Island in the 1970s the *Lone Star tick-like Lyme Disease is now spread throughout New York, New Jersey, and Connecticut*.

How could that southern species of tick get there other than through biogerm testing corruption?

Then, notes Doyle, "How did this happen?" It's occurrence can be explained largely by going through archived US government files, including those which reveal the role of globalist operative Erich Traub. She reveals:

> More pieces of evidence on the tantalizing trail of evidence pointing to a possible Plum Island/Traub/Lyme disease link: "Erich

> Traub had been working for the American biological warfare program *from his 1949 Soviet escape until 1953*...he consulted with Fort Dietrick scientists and CIA operatives...he worked for the USDA...and (in 1952) he spoke *regularly with Plum Island director Doc Shahan*. Traub can be physically placed on Plum Island at least three times-on dedication day in 1956 and two visits, once in 1957 and again in the spring of 1958. Shahan, who enforced an *ultrastrict policy against outside visitors*, each time received *special clearance from the State Department to allow Traub on Plum Island soil*."
>
> If, in fact, Traub was involved with research on Plum Island, this development would have been consistent with programs being conducted at that time involving experimentation on unwitting American citizens with biological and chemical warfare research agents: "Research unearthed three USDA files from the vault of the National Archives-two were labeled TICK RESEARCH and a third E. TRAUB. All three folders were empty. The caked-on dust confirms the file boxes hadn't been open since the moment before they were taped shut in the 1950s. Preposterous as it sounds, clandestine outdoor germ warfare trials were almost routine during this period. In 1952 the Joint Chiefs of Staff called for a vigorous, well-planned, large-scale (biological warfare) test to the Secretary of Defense later that year. It was stated, "Steps should be taken to make certain that adequate facilities are available, including those at Fort Detrick, Dugway Proving Ground, Fort Terry (Plum Island) and an island field testing area." Was Plum Island the island field testing area? Indeed, when the Army first scouted Plum Island for its Cold War designs, they *charted wind speeds and direction and found that, much to their liking, the prevailing winds blew out to sea*.

In addition, there is the following memo that was unearthed, which gives strong substance to the claim that the germ warfare facility is, in fact, the source of the pandemic:

"...The lab chief [Dr. Charles Mebus] failed to mention that Plum Island also worked on 'hard ticks,' a crucial distinction. A long overlooked document, obtained from the files of an investigation by the office of former Long Island Congressman Thomas Downey, sheds new light on the second, more damning connection to Lyme disease. A USDA 1978 internal research document titled "African Swine Fever" notes that in 1975 and 1976, *contemporaneous with the strange outbreak in Old Lyme, Connecticut, 'the adult and nymphal stages of Abylomma americanum and Abylomma cajunense were..'* being researched. Of note, it is the tiny nymph borrelia which causes the Lyme syndrome. What the scientists admit to is the fact that these ticks were infected with swine fever virus, which was then infected into pigs. As a result, they claim, it was determined that the ticks could not transmit "African swine fever virus" to the pigs.

Thus, clearly, the scientists and operatives at Plum Island where at the precise time of the outbreak experimenting with ticks which were artificially infected with deadly germs. These ticks were created as potential bioweapons to be used to attack purportedly animals: the cattle of the enemy lands. Surely, this is a cover. Surely, the ultimate purpose was to use these weaponized insects on humans.

It was Ground Zero for Lyme. Plum Island is clearly implicated as the source point for the origin of these diseases—at a minimum Lyme disease and West Nile.

How do we Lyme victims feel about it, that is about the fact that our diseases, our suffering, is the result of such filthy corruption? The general sense is one of anger, real rage, and far more. That rage must be turned into action: that is action against the perpetrators. Every effort must be made to find out the real truth behind these wretched acts, just who is responsible, who decided upon the research, who funded it: who organized and orchestrated it.

Then, what precisely did happen? Were borrelia-infected ticks released purposely? Was this yet another government-endorsed secretive human experiment? Or, was it an accident. It is largely irrelevant in either case, because the consequence is the issue at large. That consequence was and is the ruination of the health of countless millions and also the causing of premature death. The number of people who have lost their lives prematurely from Lyme is unknown. Yet, it is surely in the tens of thousands.

What is the minimal action that must be taken? Regarding the Plum Island facility the action must be serious and direct. It should be crushed into smithereens, then burnt into the ground.

Chapter Nine

Neurological Lyme

It was horrid beyond belief to endure Lyme disease in its most deadliest manifestation: weaponized neuroborreliosis. Clearly, from the symptoms I experienced a brain infection had rapidly developed as well as an infection of the spinal cord. It seemed serious beyond belief; I felt like I was going to die.

The nervous system attack was clearly massive. Who knows how many billions of these cork-screw invaders were in my central nervous system at the time of the greatest degree of the attack. The symptoms that occurred during this attack were as follows:

- feeling as if I existed in another world
- loss of focus
- a vague sense as if my head was exploding
- a vague sense of the spinal column being full, as if exploding
- headache with great pressure inside the skull
- feeling as if the head and back were burning up
- panicky feeling

- stiffness of the neck
- Stiffness of the spine
- insomnia
- waking up with a neck ache
- desire to pull my hair out of my head

All these symptoms are now gone, thanks to the miracle of wild nature, that is to the aggressive therapies listed in this book. In this regard it must be noted that this applies to all Lyme disease and co-infection disease victims, not merely an isolated case. As demonstrated by Embers in his monumental work on monkeys infected with borrelia there is no hard proof that antibiotics clear the infection. Despite nearly a month of intensive drug therapy in a test done on five infected animals all such animals suffered persistence. Therefore, the only hope for seriously infested Lyme cases, whether complicated by neuroborreliosis or not, is wild spice oil therapy. In my case there is no doubt about it there would not have been such a dramatic and solid improvement in health were it not for the cures of wild nature, and the main ones that must be given credit are the super-strength form of edible oil of oregano, the multiple spice dessicated oil capsules, the wild juice of oregano, the wild turmeric oil, the wild 12:1 cat's claw, the bromelain- and papain-based antiinflammatory capsules with turmeric, along with ginger, the total body purging complex, and the deep-eezing aromatic spice oil pain rub.

Even so, at the time of the most dire circumstance it became quickly apparent what the real nature of Lyme disease is: that it is an infectious condition of the brain, spinal cord, and peripheral nerves more than any other major system, perhaps with the exception of the joints. For some reason the Lyme spirochete preferentially attacks these tissues. This may explain the rather consistent symptoms in its victims related to the brain and nervous system. The preference of the pathogen is now confirmed. The latest research indicates that the ultimate aim of the Lyme spirochete is the brain itself. After a tick or mosquito bite it only takes a mere 10 to 12 hours for this pathogen to enter the brain. Once there, if unopposed, it multiplies by the endless billions causing great destruction and decimation. In this regard it is a major cause of extremely destructive neurological conditions, including ALS and MS.

Though it has been covered before it bears repeating. Neuroborreliosis is a potentially fatal consequence of black legged, that is Lyme, tick bites.

According to G. Ramesh and cohorts publishing in the *Journal of Neuroinflammation*, 2013, Lyme neuroborreliosis is caused when the Lyme spirochete directly invades the central nervous system. This invasion affects, the investigators note, both the central part of that system, the brain and spinal cord, and also the peripheral nerves. Incredibly, the cork-screw pathogen directly corrupts the nerve fibers and cells as a result of its ability to actually invade such tissues. It truly is a bioweapon meant to disable and destroy—and what better way to do so than invade the nervous tissues. The result is nerve root inflammation and, consequently, loss of sensation, pain, and weakness and in some cases loss of motor function.

Investigations have determined that there is gross inflammation as a result of the infestation in the spinal cord, the various condensations of nerves known as ganglia, and the brain itself. The peripheral nerves also become inflamed, a condition known as radiculitis.

In monkeys infected with the germ dire consequences result. It is presumed that humans also suffer such consequences. This is actual destruction of the cells within the spinal cord and brain, known as nerve cell apoptosis. As a result of their experiments on monkeys Ramesh and his group "hypothesized that B. burgdorferi induces inflammation mediators in the glial and neurola cells and that this inflammation...*precipitates glial and neuronal cell apoptosis*." In other words, the highly toxic invasion and reactions caused by the spirochete led to such a high degree of oxidative damage that it caused gross death of nerve cells.

Nerve cells are not easy to regenerate. Thus, every effort must be made to purge the spirochete from the body in order to curtail this potentially deadly damage. Let, then, the power of the cork-screw pathogen not be taken lightly, especially considering its weaponized nature. In this regard it appears that it has been cultivated to cause the maximum degree of invasiveness. Even so, it is not the ultimate power. For all those who are afflicted with this vile germ let them never give up hope. Let them fight back with all their powers through the use of natural cures, those cures created by the great Master of the Universe for human benefit. There is surely great power in these natural medicines, far more so than any drugs and/or chemicals.

As demonstrated by Lida Mattman in her monumental book *Cell Wall Deficient Forms: Stealth Pathogens* the Lyme bacillus is found not only in patients with such conditions but also in those with a variety of other diseases. These diseases include a wide range of neurological conditions. Mattman has recovered the Lyme spirochete from not only ticks but also mosquitos, fleas, and mites. She has also found the pathogen in the urine, blood, spinal fluid, and semen of individuals diagnosed with neurological conditions. More direly, she has found it in human brain cells, living and thriving.

Studying the disease from its earliest origins she has cultured the germ from a wide range of patients and patient tissues. In 1993 she cultured *Borrelia burgdorferi* from some

43 of 47 patients with chronic neurological disease. This is definitive proof of the role of this agent in the cause of such diseases. This is confirmed by the testing in controls, where only two of 46 were culture positive.

There is no need for more proof than that. Obviously, this cork-screw pathogen is a major cause of chronic, degenerative neurological conditions.

Mattman is an expert at staining techniques where she can find the spirochete living in and infecting brain tissue. It was she who first made it clear that in chronic degenerative diseases of the brain, including ALS, MS, Alzheimer's disease, and Parkinson's disease, the spirochete is found. Her proof is compelling. In eight of eight Parkinson's disease cases the spirochete was recovered, and she has also found that in a high percentage of individuals with ALS the brain is infected. In Alzheimer's disease all the cases she has tested thus far have proven positive. The same universality is seen in multiple sclerosis, with 100% of the tested individuals proving positive. In this case Mattman was given access to actual brain tissue. Through special tissue staining techniques she discovered *live spirochetes*, infecting brain cells.

The Alzheimer's cases are particularly curious. This relates to the high incidence of this condition in takers of Premarin. Made from mare's urine, Premarin is surely infested with a wide range of germs and/or their cysts, with the Lyme spirochete likely being an infesting agent as horses are commonly attacked by ticks. Perhaps this is why the incidence of Alzheimer's disease in long-term users of this drug is so high.

It's not just the chronic neurological victims who suffer under this burden. In an assessment of 25 cases of chronic fatigue syndrome (CFS) by Mattman and her group all patients had Lyme bacillus infections. Mycoplasma species are also found in CFS patients, while it is also seen in a majority of cases of Lyme disease. The point is that Lyme-associated pathogens routinely infect the central nervous system, as well as the muscles and the joints, and thus could very well be the key cause of chronic, degenerative conditions, including chronic fatigue syndrome and fibromyalgia, typically regarded as 'cause unknown.'

As noted by Garth Nicholson in *Chronic Bacterial and Viral Infections in Neurodegenerative and Neurobehavioral Diseases,* "Infectious agents may enter the CNS (central nervous system) through infected macrophages;" noting that the Lyme bacillus readily infects such macrophages. They may also, he describes, "gain access" through a process known as "trancytosis," which means direct entry, essentially, into the brain tissue. A weakened blood-brain barrier (BBB) aids in such transfer. Exposure to toxic compounds, such as solvents and heavy metals, weaken that membrane. A heavy metal burden in the individual would add to such toxicity. In fact, heavy metals, particularly mercury and lead, damage the blood-brain barrier, increasing the potency and invasiveness of Lyme spirochete infection. Mercury is exceptionally toxic to this protective system, essentially causing the barrier to be corroded: thinned down to oblivion.The BBB is also greatly damaged as a result of alcohol consumption. Another mechanism is directly into the nerve sheaths through a phenomenon known as "intraneural transfer."

Nicholson upholds the findings of Mattman, saying that in ALS patients B. burgdorferi is commonly if not routinely found as a key perpetrator. In ALS victims in New York, he notes, some 50% of those tested for the bacteria had active infection versus only 10% of controls. This is compelling proof that nervous system infestation by the spirochete is a major cause of the disease. This proof is critical, as it guides to the necessary therapy in this standardly regarded 'incurable' syndrome. That therapy is the aggressive use of wild spice oil complexes as well as high-density (12:1) raw cat's claw powder. Regarding the spice oils it is those which have the greatest capacity for penetrating the BBB that are of greatest need. These whole food supplements include the juice of wild oregano, the multiple aromatic complex consisting of essences of rose water, orange blossom, sage, rosemary, and oregano as well as the mycelized oil of wild oregano.

No doubt, borrelia is capable of great damage to neurological tissue, but the immense degree of this damage is rarely recognized. An autopsy on a Lyme victim demonstrates the degree. This is in regard to a Japanese woman, who, apparently, contracted the disease while in the USA. Upon her return to Japan she presented with extreme signs of brain damage, so-called cerebellar signs and mental deterioration in a most acute way. Tests demonstrated elevated serum antibiotics to the spirochete. Within four years she was dead. Upon autopsy it was discovered that she had lesions throughout the brain and spinal cord, including so-called spongioform changes, that is holes in the brain like those seen in a sponge: a mad cow-like presentation.

The damage was extreme beyond comprehension. Essentially, there were punch holes throughout the brain matter, and the spinal cord suffered not only cavities but also demyelination, particularly in the thoracic region. Pathologists determined that there was massive destruction of the neurons. The immune cells of the brain, the microglia, were extensively activated, and there were actual white blood cells, lymphocytes, which had infiltrated the brain in an attempt to purge the pathogen. It was a gross case of neuroborreliosis, make no mistake about it.

In *Neurosurgery*, 1992, Lyme infection of the brain was found to manifest in yet another way. The spirochete, the investigators determined, deemed by them a "neurotrophic agent," readily attacks the central nervous system, where it may grow in an uncontrolled manner. That is precisely what it did in this case, striking a mere child. The patient had suffered for 10 years with signs and symptoms of a multiple sclerosis-like condition, with neuropathy, mental disturbances, and encephalitis-like symptoms. CT-scans established that there was a mass lesion in the brain. No one had determined at that point the cause. Then, the cause was recognized through a combination of biopsy and blood tests. It was a Lyme spirochete-induced mass. Upon diagnosis, the child was treated with antibiotics, and apparently, the neurological symptoms improved.

With deep-seated infestation of the nervous system there is needed a multi-phasic approach necessary to root the spirochete out of all nerve tissues. Moreover, it is not sufficient to merely root them out and destroy them. The nervous system tissue must be strengthened in order to prevent further infection. Too, if it is damaged, which is likely in any case of severe, acute Lyme or chronic Lyme, then, that nerve tissue must be regenerated and healed after it is traumatized by the infectious agents and its toxins. Spirochetes kill nerve cells. They also cause a kind of damage known as amyloid formation, a phenomenon commonly seen in brains of those with Alzheimer's disease. Amyloid is a toxic pigment, and its presence is a sign of nerve cell degeneration. Those nerve cells tainted with the pigment must be cleansed, revived, and regenerated for the ultimate cure to be achieved.

It cannot be over-emphasized. For the reversal of virtually impossible to cure, that is medically, conditions such as Alzheimer's disease, ALS, and Parkinson's disease, spice oils and their aromatic spice waters are invaluable. They help halt the production of amyloid pigment while also aiding it in purging. Other natural medicines which assist in this regard are wild, raw chaga sublingual drops, red sour grape powder, wild cat's claw, and wild turmeric.

There are certain nutrients which are key for protecting the blood-brain barrier and also the nerve cells themselves. These nutrients include raw, whole food cholesterol, that is the kind of cholesterol found in raw eggs, natural-source resveratrol from grapes, as found in red sour grape powder, whole food, unprocessed omega 3 fatty acids, as found in, for instance, fatty salmon oil derived from the brains and head tissues of wild salmon, as well as burbot liver extract, thymoquinone, a substance found in black seed oil, whole food B complex, and wild-source, naturally occurring vitamins A and D. Such substances and/or whole food complexes are highly aggressive in both protecting the blood-brain barrier from degeneration as well as inducing regeneration. Wild chaga is also a key complex for preventing nerve cell degeneration as well as for rebuilding such cells and also the blood-brain barrier. It is the raw chaga extracts which have the greatest power in this regard such as the spice oil-based raw sublingual drops or raw, wild chaga–birch bark capsules.

Clearly, according to the available data the spirochetes cause cell death in nerve organs. That leads to great toxicity, as mentioned in part because of the deposition of amyloid pigment. To protect the brain against Lyme invasion it is necessary to clear all toxins, especially those which damage the blood-brain barrier. In particular, all efforts should be made to purge mercurial toxins from the body. An ideal formula for doing so is the complex substance, total body purging agent. Another agent for purging this is wild dandelion, root in the form of a tea combined with wild chaga. Such formulas greatly increase the production of bile, purging mercury, as well as lead, from the liver, and ultimately, other tissues. Regarding amyloid formation, wild chaga, in particular, is effective in reversing it, especially in the raw oregano-infused forms (chaga-wild oregano capsules and raw, wild chaga sublingual drops).

Regardless, it must be presumed in the case of destructive neurological conditions that infection plays a key role, not merely by the Lyme spirochete but by other cork-screw germs, including those related to syphilis. Fungi also readily infest the brain, as do a wide range of viruses. Regarding the latter it is well established that a variety of herpetic viruses are primary causative agents in multiple sclerosis. Other germs which readily infect the nervous tissue include chlamydia, mycoplasma, amebas, encephalitic viruses, and meningococci.

The symptoms attributable to spirochete infection of the brain are vast as well as diverse. Such symptoms include severe headache, a heavy sensation in the head, visual disturbances, including visual loss, optic neuritis, depression, anxiety, compulsiveness, agitation, fits of rage, numbness of the extremities, foot drop, loss of muscle strength in the arms and shoulders, stiffness of the neck, memory loss, excessive sensitivity to sound, blurry vision, insomnia, and mental confusion. Additionally, some people suffer from numbness or hypersensitivity of the joint reflexes, sensitivity abnormalities in the fingertips, excessive heat sensations, muscle twitching, tics, and abnormal sweat patterns. There may also be direr symptoms such as slurring of the speech, loss of coordination, seizures, partial paralysis, or even as stated previously total paralysis of an entire side of the body.

In this regard the germ causes great inflammation within the brain and spinal cord. It may also cause an inflammatory reaction in the cranial nerves, including the facial nerve through which explains its relationship to the cause of Bell's palsy.

When it attacks other cranial nerves, there may be novel symptoms. Such symptoms include blurry vision, double vision, dizziness, hearing loss, tinnitus, drooping of the eyelid (ptosis), and numbness, pain, and/or tingling of the face.

The great challenge is in relation to the structure of the germ. Because of its cork-screw powers it can readily invade the brain, burrowing right through the blood-brain barrier. Once within the brain tissue it frequently mutates into a cell wall-deficient form, and through this form it evades the immune system. It also has the capacity, as a result of its immune neutralizing powers, to persist in the nervous system. Microscopic imagery shows it actually living in the nerve cells, where it produces great toxicity. Ultimately, as mentioned previously in many instances it kills these nerve cells. When it kills such cells, it produces great corruption, adding to the toxic, noxious burden on the brain and spinal cord. The toxins accumulate to such a degree that these, too, cause nerve cell fatality.

That the Lyme spirochete flourishes in the brain and spinal cord long after the tick bite is beyond dispute. It actually hides there, inside the cells but also in the brain fluids. In people with Lyme-related neurological symptoms surely it is there, infecting and even destroying these tissues. Consider an analysis by J. Miklossy on chronic or "late-stage" neuroborreliosis. Notes Miklossy, the great danger is in the fact that borrelia is able to "evade...destruction by the host immune reactions," and therefore, "persist in host tissues." As a result, it causes sustained "chronic infection and inflammation." Therefore, if neuroglical symptoms arise in a person with a known tick bite, this is a sign that the organism is infesting the nervous system.

Regarding neuroborreliosis, it is not likely that the pathogen will exit the brain tissue without being forced out: without being categorically killed. At first, commonly, the spirochete infects the brain stem. This can be highly dangerous, as this region of the brain exerts great powers over the muscular system as well as the critical organ systems. The zone of danger is vast and the risks are extreme. At any moment the Lyme infection may proceed to a potentially deadly neurological condition, which may be seemingly irreversible.

Thus, aggressive action must be taken, using the oil of wild oregano internally and topically, while also taking the juice of wild oregano internally. Regarding topical application the oil may be used on the areas of the disease process. This means rubbing it on the scalp and base of the head. It also means rubbing it about the ears and even on the ears. Also, the oil can be rubbed up and down the spine. It should create a burning sensation if this is done correctly. The deep-eezing multiple spice oil complex can also be rubbed in such a manner. Too, the water soluble type of wild oregano oil, the emulsified type, can be added directly into the ear.

Topical treatment is often an essential part of the protocol. Through this method the spice oils can have direct access to the body and systems through the lymph. It may offer the hope for the cure when all other therapies fail. Immediately after a tick bite, in fact, within hours the spirochetes find access to both the brain and spinal cord, where they thrive. Infection of these critical tissues may develop within a mere 12 hours after the bite. This accounts for the syndrome of sudden tick bite paralysis that occurs in many people, and not just from a Lyme tick bite; in other words, a wide range of other ticks may cause this. In this regard the infection resembles neurosyphilis. Too, like neurosyphilis the Lyme infestation may remain dormant, only to become revived months or years after the initial infection. Stress is a major factor in causing such a revival. Therefore, every effort must be made to keep psychic stress to a minimum.

It is a dire circumstance, that is for such a vigorous pathogen to actively infect the brain and associated tissues. In this regard it should be recognized that the spirochete literally consumes brain cells as food. If nothing is done, in all likelihood the infestation will worsen, leading to a progression in the disease. Untreated Lyme can result in actual neurological disease as previously indicated such as ALS, multiple sclerosis, Parkinson's disease, seizure syndromes, and Alzheimer's disease as well as neuropsychiatric disorders, including paranoia, obsessive-compulsive disorder, severe anxiety, and schizophrenia. The untreated infection in the brainstem and other neurological systems can even lead to deafness and blindness. It can even cause stroke.

Consider the following case history. A 56-year-old woman contracted Lyme disease which was diagnosed early. She was placed on a prolonged course of antibiotics. Some 18 months after the conclusion of antibiotic therapy she presented with complete paralysis of her facial muscles. It was documented that the patient suffered from neuroborreliosis and the final diagnosis was borrelia-induced stroke.

No chances can be taken with this disease. It must be treated aggressively and decisively to be obliterated from the body. The spice oil-based natural medicines are the most potent of all naturally occurring substances in that regard. They are greatly superior to antibiotics and far safer, as the aforementioned case history demonstrated.

Regarding the persistence of the organism in the brains of tick bite victims it was Alan MacDonald, M.D., who made the connection. Studying the link between Lyme disease and Alzheimer's patients what he found was no surprise, since the Lyme spirochete has a great preference for brain and nerve tissue. As reported by Guardianlv.com, "MacDonald grew Lyme spirochetes from Alzheimer's brains..." That brain tissue was taken from various pathology banks.

He attempted to publish his findings as a major research article. That was blocked by the American Medical association, which did not want to publish it, so the organization claimed, under the guise, incredibly that it would "provoke public concern and anxiety." He was finally able to publish his findings as a letter to the editor, titled "Borrelia in the brains of patients *dying of dementia*, 1986." All this time a key element revealing the danger of this disease was known, but it was fully suppressed. As a result, nothing was done about it.

The neurotoxins of Lyme

It is not merely the infestation that is at issue. The wretched germ produces a wide range of neurotoxins, which greatly disrupt neurological function. These toxins disrupt the function of nerve cells, causing them to, essentially, shrivel up and die. Moreover, it is capable of causing fatality, even from strokes as well as total body paralysis, as is seen in ALS. In this regard a review of certain case histories is crucial to demonstrate the degree of damage and suffering it inflicts upon people. According to one Lyme sufferer, posting on the Internet:

> I just want to know if anyone else has gone through or is going through what I am (going through). I have never felt so horrible in

> my entire life. There is nothing like it. The "symptoms" are agonizing. I do not even feel like the same person (essentially) feeling out of it, headache, warp in the head, dizzy, sound sensitive, complete stress and anxiety that ultimately turn to overwhelming panic and sinking feelings.
>
> There is also "brain fog" or "memory problems;" that is an understatement. It is more like feeling like half your brain is missing, not even how human consciousness should feel, detached, unreal, surreal, emotions on a total roller coaster.

This is likely the result of the noxious effects of Lyme spirochete toxins on the nerve cells. It also likely the consequence of Candida toxins, as this person was on long-term IV antibiotics. Candida overload would likely account for the brain fog. The symptoms are well established in this fungal overload syndrome and are also a result of the invasion of massive numbers of spirochetes into the brain cells.

Protocol for nervous system Lyme infection

Whether ALS, multiple sclerosis, Parkinson's disease, Alzheimer's disease, or hard-core chronic Lyme it is irrelevant. It's the same protocol for all, although with active Lyme disease it may be necessary to be extra aggressive in the dosing.

Supplements/Dosages for moderate cases of neurological degeneration due to Lyme bacillus infestation:

- wild oil of oregano as sublingual drops, 20 drops three times daily
- juice of wild oregano (crosses the blood-brain barrier readily): one ounce twice daily
- multiple aromatic spice essence consisting of essences of

rose, orange blossom, rosemary, sage, and oregano: one or more ounces daily

- mycelized oil of wild oregano: 20 or more drops twice daily (readily crosses the blood-brain barrier)
- cold-extracted wild oil of oregano with wild bay leaf oil and black seed oil as sublingual drops: 20 or more drops twice daily
- wild, raw purple grape extract plus muscadine grape skin extract: 2 or more tablespoonsful daily
- wild, raw turmeric extract, ideally as sublingual drops: 50 to 100 drops twice daily
- Super Cat's Claw Concentrate (12:1 concentrate), available at Americanwildfoods.com: one teaspoonful or more daily or twice daily in juice or smoothies (start slowly on this and work up, like a half teaspoonful daily)
- the yolks of three to four raw organic eggs, taken each morning as is or in a smoothie on an empty stomach

Dosages/supplements for severe to extreme cases of neurological degeneration due to Lyme bacillus infestation, including those complicated by intoxication with heavy metals:

- wild oil of oregano as sublingual drops: 40 drops three or more times daily
- juice of wild oregano (crosses the blood-brain barrier readily): one or more ounces twice daily
- aromatic multiple essence complex consisting of essences of rose, orange blossom, sage, rosemary, and oregano: two or more ounces twice daily
- mycelized oil of wild oregano: 40 or more drops twice daily

(readily crosses the blood-brain barrier)

- wild, raw purple grape extract plus muscadine grape skin extract: 2 or more tablespoonsful daily
- wild, raw turmeric extract, ideally as sublingual drops: 100 drops three times daily
- Super Cat's Claw Concentrate (12:1 concentrate): two teaspoonfuls or more daily in juice or smoothies
- fatty wild salmon oil rich in unprocessed omega 3 fatty acids, along with vitamins A and D: 6 or more capsules twice daily
- whole food B complex powder made from rice bran concentrate, heat-killed torula yeast, and royal jelly: two tablespoonsful daily
- total body purging agent, as a 12-oz liquid: one ounce twice daily
- wild, raw teasel root as a natural non-alcoholic extract: 8 to 10 drops daily
- wild dandelion–chaga tea: 2 cups daily
- wild, raw chaga sublingual drops: 50 drops twice daily
- the yolks of three raw organic eggs, taken each morning on an empty stomach or in a smoothie.

Topical treatment

For the treatment of nervous system infestation by the Lyme spirochete the wild oil of oregano is most versatile. The ideal type to use is the higher strength form, which has a greater dosage of oregano oil per the extra virgin olive oil emulsion. The method of topical treatment is as follows:

- rub the oil of oregano and/or the deep-eezing multiple spice oil up and down the spinal column in goodly amounts; let it set there, while resting for a few minutes; leave it on and carry on with the day

- do another rub at night, same procedure
- rub the oil on the shins vigorously; the shins have lymphatic ducts that are right next to the skin, between the skin layer and the bone; through this superficial connection the oil can be taken up into the lymphatic system, where it can then be distributed to act against the spirochete
- rub the soles of the feet, especially at night; put socks on and sleep with the oil rub; this will aid against Lyme-induced insomnia

Other topical agents

Other topical agents/formulas that are useful in neurological Lyme include the bone activating complex of oils of wild rosemary, sage, and oregano, and wild chaga tissue-healing cream. The deep-eezing multiple spice rubbing oil has already been mentioned. Like the bone-activating rubbing oil it is highly effective. All such formulas can be rubbed up and down the spine and on any involved area.

These are exceedingly powerful protocols, which will greatly aid in the battle against the Lyme bacillus. Simultaneously, the natural supplement complexes in these protocols will assist in the purging of any co-infections, including those by babesia, mycoplasma, bartonella, and ehrlichia. The point is to never give up regardless of the degree of the infestation. No doubt, natural medicines are the answer for a long-term cure. It may take weeks or months to achieve it. Yet, if people stay the course through the power of wild nature, they will achieve the ultimate result, which is the elimination of the Lyme bacillus and other tick-borne germs from the tissues. Once it is completely eliminated, then, a cure can be achieved. There is no other option. Antibiotics are not the answer for such a complex disease which may be caused by a multitude of factors. These factors include a multiplicity of infectious agents, including those agents which cannot be killed with drugs, poor nutrition, lack of healthy exercise, and stress. All must be dealt with adequately in order for the Lyme-based or other cause-based neurological disorders to be resolved.

Side effects of natural cures?

While there is no toxicity to the natural remedies described in this book, no possibility of, for instance, liver or kidney damage, there is one issue. This is the occurrence of reactions related to the positive aspects of spice oils and their complexes. It's specifically related to their killing and cleansing powers. Obviously, for instance, if countless billions of germs are suddenly killed, toxins will be produced. Too, as a result of the mobilization of various poisons and toxins there could be a toxicity of sorts. This happens as the poisons are released and/or mobilized.

A reaction can occur, known as a cleansing reaction or detox response. There is even a well-established medical term for side consequences of cleansing, known as a Herxheimer response.

In fact, in a short time many billions of germs can be killed. The poisons from these germs can be spilled into the body, including rather potent ones known as endotoxins. This is not a big issue, though, with the spice oils, especially the oil of wild oregano but also cumin oil. These oils destroy endotoxins aggressively. Even so, regarding the Herxheimer response there are certain possible signs and symptoms. These signs and symptoms of a detoxification response include joint and muscle aches, hives, rashes, fatigue, bone aches, flu-like symptoms, mental fog, headache, dizziness, irritability, nausea, diarrhea, bloating, swollen glands, numbness, a sensation of feeling toxic, as if 'dying,' itchy skin, swollen throat, congestion, joint swelling/pain, and the development of blotches on the skin.

A point needs to be emphasized. None of these reactions are dangerous. In fact, the Herxheimer reaction is an established medical consequence, that is a result of antibiotic use. It was published long ago that in certain infectious bacterial diseases, including Lyme and TB, upon the administration of antibiotics Herxheimer/cleansing responses are to be expected. They have never been regarded as a toxic consequence. They are also seen in African tick relapsing fever.

In Lyme disease Herxheimer is a real, undeniable issue, especially in relation to germ-killing. Both antibiotics and natural germ killers can induce such a reaction. It is to be expected. As the germs are being killed and neutralized toxins can be produced. As a rule, people who develop these reactions are no worse off than before it occurred. That's because the Herxheimer response is a healing reaction, essentially a positive sign.

It is tempting for some to cut back on those agents which induce this response. This is inappropriate; a person should forge through it by increasing the intake of the Herxheimer-inducing substances. Even so, there are a few extra-potent supplements that can defeat Herxheimer reactions. These include the following whole food and wild-source supplements:

- whole crude wild oregano herb with *Rhus coriaria*, organic onion, and organic garlic
- wild, raw dandelion leaf and root extract
- deep-eezing multiple spice rubbing oil

- total body purging agent
- wild oil of turmeric
- Inflammation-eezing bromelain and papain enzyme supplement with ginger and organic turmeric
- oil of wild oregano (food-grade, edible, mountain-grown)
- wild yarrow tea
- wild hyssop tea
- wild chaga/birch bark tea

Is a tick on? What to do (in review)

It is useful to review just what to do if a tick is found on the body. Ideally, the insect should be super-saturated with a triple or super-strength oil of wild oregano. Also, any oil which contains cinnamon, bay leaf, and/or sage will also destroy ticks. It is easier and safer to remove the tick if it is dead. When it is dead, adhere to the following instructions: With a tweezer grasp the tick as close to skin as possible. Then, gently pull upward. Never twist or torque it; keep it in an even plane. Too, never grasp in on its belly; get down to the skin as close to the head as possible. Then, remove it gently. After doing so, disinfect the site through applying the spice oils. Ideally, saturate a bit of cotton with the oil, and tape it on the area. Leave this on for 24 hours.

Keep the tick in rubbing alcohol, if desired. Record the date of recovery.

The tick can be pulled out alive if it is just barely attached. If its deeply entrenched, though, this cannot be done. It must be killed first by the spice oils. Then, it can be safely removed.

Chapter Ten

Natural Cures to the Rescue

The fact that Lyme disease is reversible through the use of natural cures is surely the most fantastic news conceivable. In this regard this disease and its associated conditions are needlessly destroying the health of countless millions of people yearly. Something has to be done. Antibiotics alone are only a part of the answer.

It is categorically true. Millions of new cases of Lyme disease occur yearly. There is no other medical condition which can compare to its capacity to corrupt the health of people where they have no means of self-defense, other than, of course, avoiding the bite. Besides the established drugs these teeming millions of victims have few if any options. If the antibiotics fail, then, what are they to do?

Through a wide range of natural complexes the battle against Lyme can be won in virtually all cases. Regardless, the body—the immune system—needs assistance in waging this war. In this regard dramatic improvement, the very result that all victims desire, will not happen by chance. It also will not in many cases result from orthodox treatment alone. Without the wild oregano oil therapy, along with adjunctive spice oil natural medicines, there is no possibility that a sense of normalcy would have returned *regarding my health.* Despite the dire threat at hand a cure was achieved. The spice oil-based natural medicines described, here, plus the various adjunctive natural remedies, saved my life. They will save the lives of countless others, too, if they are used judiciously.

Full list of anti-Lyme remedies

It is worthy to, once again, review all the natural medicines listed in this book. People are interested in exact protocols, understandably so. Regardless, because of the difficulty in fully eradicating Lyme disease the broadest level of natural medicines will be described. Only the most potent natural medicines are worthy of such a description. Most of these substances serve the purpose of eradicating the Lyme spirochete and other tick-borne germs. These substances also act to purge and/or destroy those toxins which are produced by the germ. In contrast, by no means can antibiotics do so. In fact, they routinely add to the burden of microbial toxins in the body, being drugs derived from microbes themselves. There is also the benefit from natural cures of regeneration, as Lyme and its co-infecting agents cause great tissue destruction, including the destruction of joint linings and muscular tissue. There are no drugs which offer such powers, which can assist in the rebuilding and regeneration of tissue. Only natural substances do this.

Regarding the various co-infections, along with infestations by parasites, the supplements also effectively assist in the destruction of such agents. In addition, certain of these natural medicines offer antiinflammatory powers and also certain powers to stimulate the healing of damaged tissue.

The human body cannot withstand the burden of a multiplicity of pathogenic infections. Nor can it handle the overwhelming toxicity of multiple drug therapy, that is the use of a multiplicity of drugs for numerous infections. The use of a wide range of natural cures, though, is comparatively harmless, and there are no major interactions to be concerned with, unlike drugs. In fact, the natural medicines mentioned here have the highly sought-after positive effect of enhancing the efficacy of any anti-Lyme drugs.

Even so, the number of supplements may prove overwhelming to many. Partly, this is the result of financial issues. Many people have no means to purchase all such listed supplements. The quality is exceptional, and so is, therefore, the cost. Thus, there will be an attempt to prioritize for those who have budgetary concerns.

The full list of key supplements in the battle against Lyme and all co-infection syndromes is as follows:

- inflammation-easing enzyme complex with bromelain and papain
- oil of wild oregano (food-grade, edible, mountain-grown) the one that is safe for daily use
- multiple spice oil complex consisting of dried or dessicated oils of oregano, cumin, sage, and cinnamon
- raw, wild CO_2 (supercritical) oregano oil as sublingual drops
- juice of wild oregano
- mycelized oil of wild oregano
- inflammation-easing deep-eez multiple spice oil complex (highly potent)

- wild oil of turmeric as capsules or sublingual drops
- wild Super-Cat's Claw concentrate (12:1)
- raw, wild chaga capsules and/or emulsion
- wild-based multiple aromatic essence complex consisting of essences of rose petals, orange blossoms, sage, rosemary, and oregano
- wild, raw naturally extracted teasel root extract
- natural multiple vitamin whole food complex as a pack of pills and capsules
- natural whole food vitamin C, as either capsules or powder (camu camu and acerola based)
- wild, raw dandelion root plus greens extract
- wild, raw total body purging complex as a 12-ounce bottle
- wild fish oil complex as a steam-distilled, unrefined complex made from wild sockeye salmon
- healthy bacterial supplement, ideally Ecologic 500 based
- wild, raw baobab powder
- red sour grape powder
- natural whole food B complex powder
- wild dried hibiscus flower tea
- wild yarrow tea
- village-made Mediterranean pomegranate syrup
- natural whole food protein powder from sprouted brown rice and hemp powders
- wild dandelion root and chaga tea
- wild chaga healing cream (beeswax base)

Extremely basic anti-Lyme plan

The basic anti-Lyme plan is an effective one and may be useful for the majority of cases. This basic plan is simply to use the oil of wild oregano, edible, mountain-grown type (beware of cheap imitations; to do this therapy only the edible, wild spice form can be used daily). The protocol is as follows:

- oil of wild oregano as sublingual drops or drops in juice/water: 20 or more drops twice daily; also use topically
- whole crude wild oregano herb with *Rhus coriaria*, organic onion, and organic garlic: 3 caps twice daily

Basic anti-Lyme supplement plan

With the moderate plan the multiple spice extract, along with the juice of oregano, is added, along with a probiotic. This is necessary for any case which is persistent, that is chronic:

- oil of wild oregano: 30 or more drops 3 times daily
- multiple spice oil capsules: 3 caps twice daily
- juice of wild oregano: one ounce twice daily
- Ecologic 500 based probiotic supplement: 2 tsp. at night
- whole crude wild oregano herb with *Rhus coriaria*, organic onion, and organic garlic: 4 caps twice daily

Moderate-to-severe anti-Lyme supplement plan

- oil of wild oregano: 40 drops 3 times daily
- multiple spice oil capsules: 3 caps 3 times daily
- juice of wild oregano: 2 ounces 2 times daily
- Wild Peruvian Amazon Super Cat's Claw (12:1): one tsp.
- HealthBAC Ecologic 500-based probiotic supplement:

3 tsp. 2 times daily

- total body purging agent: one ounce or more daily
- wild oil of turmeric: 40 drops 2 times daily
- natural whole food vitamin complex as a daily 'pak' of pills: one pak
- wild greens flushing agent (as drops under the tongue): 40 drops
- wild dandelion root and chaga tea: one cup
- deep-eezing multiple spice rubbing oil: as needed
- whole crude wild oregano herb with *Rhus coriaria*, organic onion, and organic garlic: 6 caps twice daily
- wild, raw naturally extracted teasel root extract: 8 to 10 drops daily
- bone activating wild sage, rosemary, and oregano capsules plus MCHC: 2 caps twice daily

Severe-to-extreme anti-Lyme supplement plan

- oil of wild oregano: 50 drops 3 times daily
- multiple spice oil capsules: 3 caps 4 times daily
- juice of wild oregano: 2 oz. 2 times daily
- Wild Peruvian Amazon Super Cat's Claw (12:1): one tsp. 2 times daily
- Ecologic 500 based probiotic supplement: 3 tsp.
- total body purging agent: one oz. 2 times daily
- wild oil of turmeric: 100 drops 2 times daily
- natural whole food vitamin complex as a daily 'pak' of pills: 2 paks

- whole food B complex powder: 2 T.
- special supplement for adrenal support known as Body Shape Diet Adrenal-Type formula: 3 caps 2 times daily
- wild greens flushing agent (as drops under the tongue): 80 drops
- whole crude wild oregano herb with *Rhus coriaria*, organic onion, and organic garlic: 8 caps twice daily
- wild dandelion root and chaga tea: 2 cups
- deep-eezing multiple spice rubbing oil: as needed
- wild chaga healing cream (beeswax base): rub on any inflammed, swollen, or irritated area.
- wild, raw naturally extracted teasel root extract: 10 to 12 drops daily
- fat soluble vitamin-rich raw freshwater cod liver oil complex (Omega-ADK): 1 tsp. or more daily
- bone activating wild sage, rosemary, and oregano capsules plus MCHC: 3 caps twice daily

Extreme-plus anti-Lyme supplement plan

- oil of wild oregano: 80 drops 3 times daily
- multiple spice oil capsules: 3 caps 5 times daily
- juice of wild oregano: 2 oz. 2 times daily
- Wild Peruvian Amazon Super Cat's Claw (12:1): one tsp. 2 times daily
- Ecologic 500 based probiotic supplement: 3 tsp.
- total body purging agent: 2 oz. 2 times daily
- wild oil of turmeric: 100 drops 2 times daily

- natural whole food vitamin complex as a daily 'pak' of pills: 2 paks
- wild sockeye salmon oil (natural source of vitamins A & D): 8 caps daily
- whole food B complex powder: 3 T.
- special supplement for adrenal support known as Body Shape Diet Adrenal-Type formula: 3 caps 2 times daily
- wild greens flushing agent (as drops under the tongue): 100 drops daily
- wild dandelion root and chaga tea: 3 cups
- deep-eezing multiple spice rubbing oil: as needed
- whole crude wild oregano herb with *Rhus coriaria*, organic onion, and organic garlic: 8 caps twice daily
- raw, wild super critical oregano oil, as sublingual drops: 40 drops twice daily
- wild chaga healing cream (beeswax base): rub on any inflammed, swollen, or irritated area.
- wild, raw naturally extracted teasel root extract: 12 to 14 drops daily
- a fat soluble vitamin-rich raw freshwater cod liver oil complex (Omega-ADK): 2 tsp. or more daily
- bone activating wild sage, rosemary, and oregano capsules plus MCHC: 4 caps twice daily

Profoundly, exceptionally extreme anti-Lyme supplement plan

- oil of wild oregano: 100 drops 4 or 5 times daily
- multiple spice oil capsules: 3 caps 4 times daily

- juice of wild oregano: 2 oz. 2 times daily
- Wild Peruvian Amazon Super Cat's Claw (12:1): one tsp. 2 times daily
- Ecologic 500 based probiotic supplement: 3 tsp.
- total body purging agent: 2 oz. 2 times daily
- wild oil of turmeric: 100 drops 2 times daily: also use as an application or rub on diseased, inflammed, or painful joints and also areas of nerve inflammation.
- wild sockeye salmon oil (natural source of vitamins A & D): 12 caps daily
- natural whole food vitamin complex as a daily 'pak' of pills: 2 paks
- whole food B complex powder: 3 T.
- special supplement for adrenal support known as Body Shape Diet Adrenal-Type formula: 3 caps 2 times daily
- wild greens flushing agent (as drops under the tongue): 150 drops
- whole crude wild oregano herb with *Rhus coriaria*, organic onion, and organic garlic: 8 caps twice daily
- wild dandelion root and chaga tea: 3 cups
- deep-eezing multiple spice rubbing oil: as needed
- raw, wild super critical oregano oil, as sublingual drops: 40 drops twice daily
- wild chaga healing cream (beeswax base); rub on any inflammed, swollen, or irritated area.
- wild, raw naturally extracted teasel root extract: 14 to 16 drops daily

- a fat soluble vitamin-rich raw freshwater cod liver oil complex (Omega-ADK): 3 tsp. or more daily
- bone activating wild sage, rosemary, and oregano capsules plus MCHC: 5 caps twice daily

Special supplements for cardiac Lyme

- red sour grape powder
- wild, raw purple grape extract plus muscadine skin extract
- village-made Mediterranean pomegranate syrup
- wild dried hibiscus tea
- juice of wild oregano
- oil of wild oregano
- fatty sockeye salmon oil rich in vitamins A and D
- whole food vitamin complex as a single 'pak' daily
- special supplement for thyroid support, known as Body Shape Diet Thyroid-Type capsules
- wild, raw chaga sublingual drops (water, not alcohol extract)

Special supplements which can be added for neuroborreliosis

- whole food B complex powder consisting of rice bran, torula yeast, and royal jelly
- whole food-based royal jelly complex with wild rosemary and sage
- whole food-based wild vitamin C complex consisting of wild camu camu, acerola, and rose hips
- special supplement for adrenal support known as Body Shape Diet Adrenal-Type formula

- wild sockeye salmon oil (rich in vitamins A & D)

Special supplements for fighting weight loss associated with Lyme

- whole food B complex powder consisting of rice bran, torula yeast, and royal jelly
- whole food-based royal jelly complex with wild rosemary and sage
- raw royal jelly paste in Austrian pumpkin seed oil
- whole food raw protein powder consisting of sprouted brown rice, raw hemp, wild chaga, and raw yacon powder
- wild, raw oregano honey
- whole food organic sprouted brown rice, hemp, and wild chaga protein powder
- whole food vitamin complex as a daily 'pak'

Wild greens: maintenance factor-plus

For all people freshly grown dark leafy greens are essential. In all cases of chronic disease such leafy greens play a major role in recovery as well as prevention, although it should be kept in mind that the wild forms are the most potent.

In the 1930s a highly respected English physician Robert McCarrison wrote a book about nutritional deficiencies in relation to dietary practices. In this book, *Studies in Deficiency Disease,* he described a number of foods which, when eaten regularly, appeared to protect against degenerative diseases. One such food was fresh, raw greens. These were not just any kind of green vegetable but, rather, fresh, leafy greens, the kinds that grow fast and readily in late spring and early summer. Such leafy greens include lettuce of all kinds, kale, collards, arugula, mustard greens, turnip greens, beet greens, and spinach. Per McCarrison's work it was only these types of greens which offered universally protective effects, largely because of their dense supply of whole food vitamins, notably vitamins B and C.

Wild greens are even more potent in protecting the body than the commercial types. Their immense powers can be readily seen in nature. Surely, wild animals which feast on wild greens, such as deer, elk, moose, geese, ducks, and more are free of the types of diseases seen in humans, including arthritis, heart disease, hypertension, cancer, and neurological disorders. They are even seemingly protected more so than humans against chronic infectious disorders, including Lyme. They surely do not suffer the disease consequences from a mere single tick bite. If that was the case, all the wild animals would be dead and/or dying.

Fresh greens are a staple in the Lyme cure program as well as for regeneration. For medicinal effects or a high potency potential the wild greens are available as raw extracts. The top wild, raw fresh green formulas for Lyme sufferers to use daily are the wild, raw dandelion leaf and root extract, the total body purging agent, and the greens flushing agent as drops under the tongue. There is also the wild, raw nettles juice in a juice of oregano base. The key, here, is that all such supplements are raw. That is why they are so powerful.

Even so, it is crucial to achieve such flushing and cleansing, particularly in regard to the litany of toxins which accumulate in the body. These toxins accumulate mainly in the liver but can also congest the gall bladder and intestines. That load of toxins can greatly suppress organ function, including causing the suppression of immune function. To regularly cleanse and eliminate such poisons from the body is a key formula for the achievement of optimal health.

It cannot be done with commercial or even organic greens alone. The load is too great. The bioactive ingredients in farm-raised food are too low to achieve the purge. Rather, it is the wild greens which have the much sought after potency to achieve this. Moreover, they do so only in the raw state.

This is why to a large degree the animal kingdom is free of disease, that is since wild, raw greens are on their menu constantly. Now, of course, this refers to those animals that thrive on vegetation. Regarding such animals, focusing on those in the Northern Hemisphere, what protective greens do they eat? From personal observation it has been determined that the following are among the main wild, raw greens upon which these animals feast:

wild or commercially-grown grasses of a variety of types
wild dandelion greens
wild dandelion tops
wild chickweed
wild chicory
wild raspberry leaves
wild blackberry leaves
wild strawberry leaves
wild burdock leaves (early immature growth)
wild lamb's quarters
wild sorrel
wild sour dock leaves
wild violet leaves and flowers
wild poplar leaves and buds
wild birch leaves and buds

All varieties of wild greens and other matter have powerful detoxification powers. The substances in the plant foods greatly aid in the elimination processes, through both the intestinal system and the kidneys. One group of such substances is tannic acid-rich compounds. Yet another is various waxes and resins, which are highly stimulatory to the liver and gallbladder. Another category is the flavonoids, which are also decided stimulants of the detoxification process as well as digestion. So, do eat your organic and all-natural greens. Yet, also take the wild, raw greens supplements to optimize the detoxification process. Many of such wild-source foods can be found on www.americanwildfoods.com as well certain superior health food stores.

The why of cat's claw as a key therapy

The question should arise, why the emphasis on cat's claw as an additional therapeutic agent? This substance is a complex of compounds found in the inner bark of a tree growing in the Peruvian Amazon highlands, known by the locals as Uno De Gata and by the botanical name *Uncaria tomentosa*. This inner bark possesses a number of novel properties, which makes it invaluable in the treatment of Lyme and the various co-infections. Cat's claw helps bolster immune function while acting as an antiinflammatory agent. It gets its name from the claw-shaped thorns attached to the vine.

Regarding arthritis there is some clinical evidence of value. In one study it helped reduce knee pain due to osteoarthritis. It was also tested in the Lyme-like form of arthritis, that is rheumatoid arthritis. In a pilot trial on humans those patients with this condition who took the supplement had a reduction in pain within the joints versus the control group. The benefit was held due to the various chemicals in the inner bark, which includes tannins, flavonoids, sterols, and glycosides. In one human study conducted directly with 28 cases of chronic Lyme patients 85% of all patients experienced a significant improvement in their conditions. All had tested positive for borrelia infection through Western Blot blood testing. Yet, by the study's conclusion all were negative in the testing.

Other studies indicate it is of value in boosting overall immunity. Consumption of high-grade cat's claw supplements increases the production of the body's germ-fighting antibodies. It is, without doubt, a stimulant for bone marrow function. Furthermore, a number of studies have demonstrated an anti-tumor power, where cat's claw inhibits the growth of tumor cells. It has also been shown to inhibit the growth of disease-causing viruses, including the herpes virus. Furthermore, because of its rich content of phenols it possesses significant antifungal properties and is a healthy adjunct to anti-candida therapies.

It has also been shown to boost overall health of the digestive system. In this regard there is some evidence of its value in the healing of ulcerations of the stomach and intestines. It has also been found to be of value in the fight against irritable bowel syndrome and ulcerative colitis.

This demonstrates a greater degree of efficacy than many antibiotics, which in chronic Lyme produce marginal if any results. Regardless, there is a need for such a potent anti-inflammatory and immune modulating agent in Lyme, plus as is the rule, here, this is a wild-source herbal medicine. Moreover, such wild medicines offer energetic capacities to assist in the cure.

Regarding the energetic potential of cat's claw this is true only if it is 100% raw. The 12:1 cat's claw powder from the Peruvian Amazon highlands is a purely raw, unprocessed formula.

Thus, add 12:1 Amazon-source cat's claw to any wild oregano-based supplement plan for the reversal of Lyme disease. The combination creates the potency needed for the obliteration of this condition.

Some people report "die off"-like symptoms when taking this wild herb. That is understandable, as it is a potent immune enhancer. For those who might be sensitive it is a good idea to start with small doses, like a quarter teaspoonful a day or less. The 12:1 concentrate is truly potent, far more potent than commercially available brands. A small amount is reasonable for a start, working it up to as much as a half-teaspoonful or more twice daily.

If there is a surging of joint pain symptoms, simply continue the course. In such a case it might be advisable to take the concentrate in a base of apple cider vinegar, honey, and warm water, which will not only reduce any such symptomology but will also aid in the absorption. Another option is to take it mixed in extra virgin olive oil. Regardless, a "super" form of cat's claw is an essential component of a full-fledged Lyme disease cure.

Teasel root: a potential cure?

There are a number Lyme disease sufferers who have reported positive results from a root heralded in Chinese medicine. This is teasel root, a complex know to have positive effects on the musculoskeletal system. In Chinese medicine the root is also famous for another effect: the healing of damaged and fractured bones.

Over the past few decades it was surmised that extracts of the root would be of value in Lyme disease. People began using it with beneficial results. The use of the root extract for Lyme appears to originate from the work of herbalist Mathew Wood and colleagues. It was his publication The Book of Herbal Wisdom where teasel root was popularized for Lyme to such a degree that he dedicated an entire chapter to it. Through his research he learned that the Chinese word for teasel means "restore what is broken." Surely, in Lyme one 'broken' element is the sound function of the musculoskeletal system, including the bone tissue itself.

Its name is derived from the fact that it's cone flower area was once widely used in the textile industry, providing a natural comb for clean wool and also aligning/raising the nap on such fabric. Teasel's main known actions are acting as a sweating agent, a diuretic, and an antiphlogistic, which in herbal terminology means an antiinflammatory agent. Historical uses include as an aid to stomach function and in addition to a bone fracture healing complex an agent for easing pain. Yet, its main usage today is for reducing or eliminating some of the major symptoms of Lyme disease, especially those related to the muscles and joints.

Yet another source of information on teasel root comes from W. D. Storl's Healing Lyme Disease Naturally. Here is a summary of dosage information from the book. The approach is virtually homeopathic, with the recommendation of three drops three times daily. The activity of the borrelia spirochete, the authors note, peaks every month or twenty-eight days and thus the duration of dosage should be at least a month, perhaps two months, while the dose in Storl's view should be gradually decreased after the first month of therapy.

Herxheimer responses or detox reactions are a real issue with wild teasel therapy. People need to be aware of this and attempt to forge forward with the treatment regardless. Such reactions will be minimized with the use of the wide range of other supplements mentioned in this book.

Herxheimer reactions are more extreme with alcohol extracts of the herbs. A whole food, natural extract, through raw apple cider vinegar and wild oregano oil, represents a more well tolerated wild, raw teasel root extract. The use of alcohol and glycerin introduces the potential for GMO contamination, which is not seen in the cider vinegar/wild oregano extract.

Chapter Eleven

Complications and Syndromes

There are a number of severe complications which may manifest from tick bites. Critical organ systems can readily become compromised. Key organs which are routinely infested by tick-injected germs include the heart, brain, spinal cord, liver, muscle tissue, and kidneys.

Powasson encephalitis

Viruses from vermin and other wretched mammals, including the Powasson encephalitis virus, are yet another diabolical consequence of tick bites. The existence of this viral infection demonstrates that it is not merely spirochetes and a few other bacteria, along with a modicum of protozoans, that are transmitted by ticks but, rather, the full amount of infectious agents, including deadly viruses.

In fact, the potential number of germs transferred from ticks to humans is legion. No one knows for sure the exact number. For instance, there could be dozens of viruses carried by ticks. What is it that lurks in the bloodstream and internal organs of mammals upon which the ticks feed such as mice, rats, shrews, moles, chipmunks, squirrels, skunks, possums, racoons, wolves, coyotes, deer, and more? Too, dogs are commonly afflicted with ticks, as are cats. What is in the internal systems of such animals which can cause pathology in humans? Surely, the number of germs within these animals that can corrupt the human system is vast.

This demonstrates the ultimate impotency of antibiotics alone as a means of treatment. Such drugs only treat and/or attack bacteria, and certain bacteria at that. Based on the nature of tick bites and such a wide range of potential pathogens there is need for an entirely different approach. That approach is one of purging: all the tick-injected pathogens, not merely spirochetes, rickettsia, and/or protozoans. This is the means to become fully cured of Lyme and associated diseases; in fact, the full range of germs must be purged.

Let us review the latest findings on this potentially fatal disease, which is likely more common than is advertised. According to the latest reports in Saratoga County, New York, a resident contracted this virus from a deer tick, the same one that transmits Lyme. While county officials are calling it "extremely rare," surely it is plausible that it is more common than realized. People could die of an encephalitis-like presentation if no one determined the real cause or that a tick bite was associated. Even so, the investigators have made it clear that this type of tick germ is far more aggressive than even the Lyme bacillus itself, "killing 30% of those infected statewide since 2004." Plus, they found that "its victims are infected much more quickly." According to the lead disease ecologist investigating the findings, Richard Osterfeld of the Cary Institute of Ecosystem Studies (Millbrook, New York):

"With Lyme disease once you find the tick on you, you've got a day or so to remove it before it can transmit the pathogen to you, but with Powassan virus, *a tick can start transmitting the virus within 15 minutes.*"

This demonstrates the crucial value of germicide therapy, that is the use of wild oil of oregano and the multiple spice complex, in any known, or even unknown, tick bite. Unlike Lyme, there is no medical treatment for Powassan virus; doctors can address symptoms only. The virus can cause central nervous system malfunction, meningitis, and encephalitis, the latter represented by brain swelling and inflammation.

Even so, in New York State only some 17 cases of the sickness have been proven since the mid-1990s, yet the key is *proven.* In any person who develops sudden onset meningitis and/or encephalitis while living in a tick-infested zone, especially the upper northeastern seaboard, Powassan encephalitis must be considered.

Cardiac Lyme

A catastrophe of immense proportions cardiac Lyme is far more common than is realized. It is likely responsible for numerous cases of sudden cardiac death, cause unknown. It has been long known that this wretched spirochete readily infects the heart muscle cells. It has also been established that this infestation must be caught early and reversed; otherwise, it can result in fatality. Once it infects this organ it causes a condition known as "carditis" or inflammation of the heart muscle. Demonstrating the aggression of this pathogen this occurs precisely when Lyme germs enter the heart tissues. This toxic reaction can interfere with the heart's conductive capacity, leading to a condition known as "heart block."

Symptoms of Lyme-induced heart block include lightheadedness, palpitations, chest pain, and even fainting. Other symptoms might include fever and generalized aches. Fortunately, the condition only occurs in about 2% of Lyme disease cases. Yet, still, it is no minor issue. Consider the findings of CDC investigators, who in 2013 reported a horrific phenomenon: sudden cardiac deaths from Lyme. The investigators reported three cases of bizarre sudden deaths. In one case a Massachusetts resident and Lyme victim was found dead in his car. Other than the spirochete infection this person had no other previous history of major illness. In another case the person, a New York resident, experienced chest pain at home and simply collapsed, dying before reaching the hospital. The tick was acquired in this person's case when hiking. Through heart tissue analysis the borrelia infestation was confirmed, the analysis being done because of the potential for being a heart transplantation candidate. The tests were "strongly reactive" for Lyme, scoring high in all arenas. Silver staining showed spirochetes in the heart muscle.

In yet another case a Connecticut man died suddenly after collapsing. Prior to his collapse he complained of shortness of breath and anxiety, which he suffered with for a week. Oddly, he had no other symptoms. The victim lived in a heavily wooded area and was frequently exposed to ticks. He had no history of heart disease. Autopsy revealed inflammation of the heart muscle, known as myocarditis, while staining revealed numerous spirochetes in the heart muscle. It is most incredible but the Lyme spirochete is powerful enough to take out people's hearts and kill them, even though they were previously healthy and free of heart disease.

Yet, cardiac Lyme is no match for the wild oregano, especially the combination of the oil taken as sublingual drops, along with the aromatic essence. These natural spice oil extracts rapidly obliterate the Lyme from this organ, effectively saving lives.

Muscular Lyme

It's the nature of the monstrosity that it could disable an entire system as powerful as the musculoskeletal organ. Because of its tissue boring capacity, the Lyme spirochete fully has the ability to both attack and invade muscle tissue. As extensions of the muscles it is also capable of boring into tendons and also ligaments. A virtually carnivorous type of germ once inside the muscle cells it feeds on them. This leads to an entire constellation of symptoms, including muscle weakness, paralysis, pain, aching of the involved area(s), and swelling. More direly, there may also develop muscle atrophy with virtual complete loss of function of the involved muscle.

In regard to the destruction of muscle tissues there is, surely, the need for regeneration. Here, the intake of wild chaga is ideal. Chaga is rich in sterols, needed by the muscle membranes. Upon attack of the muscle fibers and cells by the spirochete the sterols are corrupted and destroyed. Extracts of chaga, then, feed the muscular tissues, inducing cell wall rebuilding. Plus, chaga has a potent capacity to reduce muscular aching and pain, which is highly common in cases of chronic Lyme infestation. Wild turmeric is another key agent for reversing the muscular sequela. Through its potent anti-inflammatory actions it helps reverse the deep elements of inflammation in such tissues, allowing regeneration.

Unless this inflammation is eliminated a number of dire consequences may result. Lyme will destroy the muscle tissue itself. It has already been described that it readily consumes nerve cells, including those in the brain and spinal cord. The muscles can no longer get their impulses as well as their nourishment. As a result, they shrivel up and die. The most glaring example of this is ALS.

Yet, equally dire is the Lyme version of this condition. Both of these diseases involve a phenomenon known was *denervation*. Essentially, denervation is the loss of nerve impulses to the muscle tissues as a result of intoxication and/or destructive damage to nerve cells, that is nerve cell death. In this regard the two conditions are so similar it is difficult to separate them. Both lead to great abnormalities in brain wave function and nerve firing, detectable on EMGs. Likewise, both can and do progress in the same way, resulting in end stage total paralysis and death. In lesser stages there may be a wide range of disconcerting symptoms, including tics, muscle fibrillations, and cramps. There can be numbness of the extremities and the tips of the toes and fingers.

The Lyme attack on the muscles may mimic other diseases. In fact, this attack is commonly misdiagnosed as fibromyalgia and dermatomyositis, that is inflammation of the dermis of the skin and the muscles. A case history demonstrates this. As reported in *Arthritis and Rheumatology*, August 1995, a 73-year-old forest owner presented with widespread erythema, muscle pain, muscle aches, and weakness of the muscles in the arms as well as legs. Doctors initially diagnosed it as dermatomyositis. However, blood tests were positive for borrelia infection. More crucially, the organism was detected through muscle biopsy; in other words, it was clearly invasively attacking muscle tissue, in fact, thriving in such tissue.

This demonstrates the value of wild oil of oregano, as well as other spice oils and spice oil complexes, such as the deep-eezing anti-Lyme oil complex, as rubbing, actually, topical scrubbing agents. It is one of the few therapies capable of addressing this dilemma. In fact, the finding of the pathogen in muscle tissue and cells explains so much about this condition. For instance, muscle wasting, known medically as atrophy, is a prominent consequence of this disease. So is a condition known as proximal muscle weakness, as described in the case history, which is weakness of the muscles of the extremities, the shoulders and arms.

Yet, it doesn't entirely discriminate. The wretched spirochete can attack a wide range of other muscular tissues. This includes the muscles of mastication, that is those that control chewing. As mentioned, the deltoid is readily attacked, but so are the biceps and muscles of the forearm. Muscles around the hip joint, as well as their tendons, may also be invaded, as can muscular tissues of the thighs and calves.

Yet, none of this should be a surprise. It has been well established, here, that one of the chief mechanisms of action of the Lyme bacillus is invasion of the deepest recesses of the body, for instance, the central nervous system, which means the brain and spinal cord. There, it causes significant inflammation, a condition in regard to the spinal cord and peripheral nerves known as mononeuritis. The condition is defined as "inflammation of a single nerve." Yet, this oversimplifies it. When the inflammation occurs, even in a single nerve sheath, it causes corruption of the entire nervous system. This is in part through stress but also oxidative damage.

The oxidative damage, as well as the infection, must both be treated in order to achieve optimal results. Even so, once nerve damage occurs, as well as outright damage to the muscles, like muscular atrophy, it will take time to heal. The healing is achieved by destroying the Lyme bacillus and also halting all oxidative damage.

It becomes clear that for a deep invader, the muscles and nerves are the ideal residence for the Lyme bacillus. The question is how to root them out and, as well, destroy them in such tissues? It is the hot spice oils which are the key in this regard, utilized both internally and topically. In fact, the edible/topical spice oils are the only absolute hope for an ultimate cure of muscular invasion by the Lyme spirochete. Other natural substances which may assist in this regard are the enzymes bromelain and papain. These enzymes improve the microcirculation to the muscle tissues, thereby aiding in the delivery of oxygen, an antagonist to borrelia growth. They also act to reduce localized inflammation, plus they have a novel property of actually attacking foreign protein, facilitating the decontamination of these proteins from the body. The intake of high-grade bromelain and papain, combined with ginger and turmeric, as capsules but not as pressed pills, is, therefore, a major adjunct to the wild oregano oil therapy. Capsules are ideal, as it is important for these enzymes to be released immediately in the stomach environment for optimal absorption.

A protocol for the treatment of muscular Lyme is as follows:

- oil of wild oregano, super-strength: 40 or more drops three times daily as sublingual drops
- oil of wild oregano, super-strength, as a topical rub: rub vigorously on any involved muscular tissue two or more times daily
- Inflam-'eezing' high grade bromelain and papain capsules with ginger and turmeric
- wild, raw chaga emulsion as sublingual drops: 100 drops twice daily

- wild, raw chaga plus birch bark in a base of wild oregano as 500 mg capsules: 3 capsules twice daily
- wild turmeric concentrate as capsules or sublingual drops: 4 capsules twice daily or 100 drops twice daily
- deep-'eezing' aromatic spice oil rub consisting of oils of wild bay leaf, rosemary, oregano, and karabash: rub vigorously into any inflamed or involved area

Note: In all cases where mega-dose therapy of wild oregano oil is taken, there should be a simultaneous intake of a healthy bacterial supplement.

The muscles are not the only tissues which are so afflicted. The skin can also suffer a kind of atrophic degeneration as a result of the infection. This is known as acrodermatitis chronic atrophicas, for the purposes here, ACA.

In a study conducted by Asbrink and his group a kind of hard proof was found of ACA being a tick-induced disease, that is a Lyme spirochetal condition. Looking at 10 patients with ACA they did discover the Lyme germ but only in a small percentage. In this regard the work of Mattman has already been discussed, where she had determined the cork-screw form to be found only relatively rarely in infected tissue. The researchers found this true; they discovered actively infecting spirochetes in only one of the patient biopsies, in this case, biopsies of the skin.

This is still highly significant. Yet, a person might ask, "What about the other nine?" The investigators, with their novel research, had an answer for this. They made a kind of antigen 'soup' from the proteins of three different species of Lyme spirochetes and reacted this against the patients' antibodies. The result was highly revealing. Of the group of patient's serum tested all reacted against the antigen. All sera from 17 ACA patients showed high antibody titers to the three antigens.

They even looked at the antigens from the syphilis germ. Seven of the 17 also reacted to this. The investigators could only make one conclusion, which is that spirochetes, including the Lyme pathogen, are the "... causative agent of this disease."

So, it is there, in one form or another, infesting the tissues. That seems to be beyond doubt. The destructive actions of the spirochetal infection against the skin can be rather severe, causing atrophy of not only that tissue but also the underlying muscle. Simultaneously, nodules readily form, in many cases along the connective tissue sheaths. Here, it should be kept in mind that the Lyme spirochete has been known to feed off of connective tissue. Regardless, it is highly destructive, as it essentially drives its way through its cork-screw-like powers into virtually any tissue, upon which it then feeds.

Too, it should be kept in mind that the skin itself is a form of connective tissue. In fact, the disease's main initial manifestation, other than single joint disease, is the well known bullseye rash, that condition being known medically as erythema migrans (EM). EM is the most common objective manifestation of Lyme disease, seen in up to 90% of all cases.

Regarding this condition it may present as a single erythematous lesion, always circular or oval or, in fact, multiples of them. In one case of a Lyme victim in Pennsylvania some seven such circular lesions were seen on the abdominal region alone.

Genital Lyme: is it real?

The fact that Lyme can be transmitted through sexual intercourse should not come as a surprise to anyone. It is, after all, a spirochetal disease, and the spirochete, for instance, as the syphilis pathogen has a long history of infecting the genital organs. If spirochetes inhabit human genitals, they will be readily transmitted.

Regarding such transmission as a means of contracting Lyme there is new data confirming that this is very real. In a study published in the *Journal of Investigative Research* it was documented that, in fact, sexual transmission of the Lyme bacillus is a catastrophic issue. In this regard, the study demonstrates, this is far more common than is realized. Evaluating actual known cases of the infection versus controls the sperm and vaginal secretions were analyzed. While as expected all the controls were negative this was not the case for those with proven Lyme infection. All the women had active spirochetal infection of their vaginal area, while with the men some 50% were infected, meaning that half of them had active infection in their seminal tubular system as well as their prostates. Live spirochetes were readily recovered in both males and females. Moreover, in the sexually active couples evaluated in the study there was a kind of hard proof of transmission that was determined. It was deemed by the researchers that the couples had "identical strains," meaning they were passing the germs between themselves.

This is a monumental discovery. It means that Lyme is, essentially, a venereal disease and this, the researchers concluded, may account for the higher than expected incidence as would be expected from tick bites alone. Diabolically, though, this seems to support the suspicion that the original Lyme agent, the one discovered in Lyme and Old Lyme, Connecticut, has all along been a form of weaponized syphilis.

Now, people are going to feel virtually oppressed about the sexual transmission issue. No one wants to contract Lyme in such a way or give it to anyone else. This brings up a key issue, which is 'What can be done about it?' Obviously, the spice oil therapy is largely the answer. Yet, what about local treatment? This also can be achieved naturally. It cannot be readily done with oil of wild oregano, because it is extremely hot. It virtually sets the genitals on fire, although with time this dissipates. More usable are the less heat-producing spice oils such as extra virgin olive oil, emulsions of wild sage, cumin, lavender, and myrtle. A combination of these oils, or their use singly, can be applied to the genitals and also placed inside the vaginal tract. Done once or twice daily this will largely lead to an eradication of any localized infection. These also can be rubbed on the male genitals to create local penetration.

This is particularly true if the Lyme spirochete is also being treated systemically. At all costs there must be an aggressive effort to purge the spirochete from such tissues. To do so it is necessary to consume a super-strength form of oil of wild oregano, edible-type, as sublingual drops or as drops in water/juice. It may also be consumed in capsule form. Additionally, the multiple spice complex must be consumed, two more capsules three times daily. In the genital regions the Lyme bacillus is a slow-growing, smoldering pathogen. It takes time and consistent effort to eradicate it from this region. Yet, it can be done. Never lose hope. It's just a matter of time before all the tick-injected germs are eradicated.

Lyme hepatitis?

The liver serves a wide range of critical functions in the body. Any compromise in such functions has wide-ranging effects on overall health. One of its many functions is the clearance of potentially dangerous microbes from the bloodstream. Vast quantities of blood perfuse this organ on a daily basis. Thus, it must have a means of defense against potential invaders. That means of defense is a specialized set of cells known as the Kuppfer cells.

These cells are strategically placed in the liver cellular system as entrapment agents. When germs pass through the liver, which is a kind of filtration system, the germs are trapped by these cells and killed. If the Kuppfer cells are overwhelmed by an excess of the germs, they are unable to kill them all and may themselves become victims of the infestation. As a result, the liver may become chronically infected, a condition known as hepatitis.

There is significant evidence to support the development of hepatitis in Lyme victims. For instance, it is well established that after a tick bite up to 25% of all Lyme cases develop at least a degree of hepatitis. Moreover, this is not just in the acute infection wherein this occurs but also the liver may be chronically infected, where the spirochete thrives in the organ continuously. Consider the work done by a team of investigators led by Canada's M. Middelveen. The group studied a patient with chronic Lyme disease who developed hepatitis. The liver syndrome happened suddenly and was manifested by a rise in liver enzyme levels. Incredibly, this occurred during vigorous antibiotic therapy. What the researchers discovered was live, thriving spirochetes in the bloodstream but also within the liver tissue itself, the latter being determined through biopsy. No other infectious agents were found. The infection caused a kind of inflammatory damage known as granulomatous hepatitis. Thus, the researchers confirmed the persistence of infection within the liver after the course of drug therapy.

Hormone insufficiency: a key factor

The entire hormone system is compromised by this disease. Notes Moorcroft, "Hormonal dysregulation" as a result of Lyme bacillus infestation is exceedingly "common." The hormones clearly affected include melatonin, progesterone, estrogen, testosterone, adrenal steroids, and thyroid hormone, in other words, virtually all the major hormonal agents known. In this regard the condition may be readily misdiagnosed as a hormonal disorder. In other words, it is possible that conditions such as adrenal exhaustion, inflammation of the thyroid, that is thyroiditis or Hashimoto's syndrome, pituitary insufficiency, ovarian cysts, endometriosis, and pituitary adenoma, may all represent Lyme disease or at least a degree of this disease.

Too, people with hormonal imbalances are often in a weaker state than the norm. Thus, in such a condition they are in a heightened vulnerability for borrelia colonization. In particular, exhaustion of the adrenal glands greatly increases the risk of the development of tick germ-based infections. Such germs which will readily attack the low adrenal individual include the Lyme spirochete, mycoplasma, ehrlichia, anaplasma, Powasson encephalitic virus, bartonella, and babesia. Regardless, such a mass of infections places a great burden on the body, and the endocrine system suffers under the brunt of it. Both the thyroid and adrenal glands are under significant stress in attempting to deal with such infectious loads.

In any acute infection the adrenal glands are placed under great pressure. They must respond to the toxic insult through the production of steroid hormones. In Lyme it is crucial to support these glands to allow them to function at the optimal level. Foods which help sustain the adrenals are those rich in fat and protein. Also, foods naturally rich in sodium, such as celery and zucchini, are supportive as are, in particular, salty snacks themselves such as salted, roasted nuts, olives, and natural-type crackers. Key supplements for supporting the adrenal glands are oil of wild rosemary, oil of wild lavender, juice of wild oregano, and royal jelly-based formulas as well as glandular based formulas consisting of dessicated gland material derived from grass-fed Argentinian and New Zealand herds.

To balance and/or strengthen the glands it is crucial to determine the specific body and metabolic type. This will establish the weak links in the hormonal system of each individual. This can be done through the book *The Body Shape Diet* (Knowledge House Publishers, same author).

Chapter Twelve

Co-Infections

Though mentioned throughout this book the co-infections are such a significant issue in tick-borne illnesses, in Lyme, in particular, that they are worthy of their own assessment. Tough cases of Lyme usually represent a multitude of infections, often including various protozoans and viruses, along with bacteria.

Ehrlichiosis

Ehrlichiosis is caused by a tiny bacteria, which invades various cells of the body. In regard to tick pathogens there are two such germs of issue, one known as ehrlichia itself and also its related germ, anaplasma. The two germs essentially are the same in terms of their mechanism of action and the diseases they cause; nevertheless, technically, they are two separate entities.

Were these germs also released as a result of human meddling? They have been long known as veterinary pathogens but only more recently, about 1986, were recognized as causing diseases in humans.

In areas of heavy tick infestation routine testing proves a significant phenomenon: up to 20% of all people have evidence of either current or former ehrlichia infection. This means that at one point the germ had infested the body. The majority of these people, though, never notice any obvious symptoms of such an infection.

The bacteria has a unique pattern. It preferentially attacks and invades certain kinds of white blood cells, known as mononuclear phagocytes. These are more commonly known as monocytes and macrophages. More rarely, the germ invades the main type of white blood cell in the body, the neutrophils. Within these cells they form tiny colonies of reproducing germs, known as morulae.

Now, make no mistake about it even though the infection normally causes only mild-to-moderate symptoms, still, it is wretched. For instance, it readily causes diseases in farm animals and even wild ones. The two main species in this regard are E. chaffeenis and E. ewingii. It is the chaffeenis species which invades mainly monocytes and is, therefore, known also as HME, while ewingii prefers to attack neutrophils, also known as granulocytes, and this explains why it is known as HGE.

Transmitted by the so-called lone star tick, this disease mainly occurs in the Southeast and Southwest. Despite this seemingly regional density documented erhlichia infections have also been found throughout other areas of North America, including Canada. Thus, clearly, a variety of ticks house the erhlichia family of pathogens. The disease most commonly strikes in the spring and summer. The main symptoms are a sudden onset of fever, combined with chills, severe headache, and muscle pains.

In one case a victim's liver enzymes soared to over 700 (SGOT and SGPT) with the norm being a mere 25 to 35. This occurred some two weeks after the bite. The victim, a middle-aged woman, took aggressive action, in this case with the super-strength form of oil of oregano. Some 100 drops were prescribed three or four times daily. The liver enzymes were normalized within two weeks.

While in most cases the disease is self-limiting, it can result in liver damage, toxicity to the brain (encephalitis), and also fatality, the latter occurring in about 3% of all cases.

There is no accepted medical treatment for erhlichiosis. This demonstrates the novel value of spice oil supplements in fighting this condition. No doubt, the oil of wild oregano and the multiple spice oil formulas are effective against this germ. Of note, the oils would be invaluable in purging and cleansing the infected white blood cells. In fact, it is known that such white blood cells readily take up the spice oil complexes, so they can use them for germ destruction. The energy vibrations in the wild oregano oil, for instance, are sensed by the white blood cells, which will sop up the oil from the blood and then use it in the effort to kill germs.

Bartonella

Bartonella is a bacteria commonly found in biting insects, particularly fleas, lice, and ticks. The key reservoir is likely rodents; however, cats are the primary secondary reservoir for the germ. A fairly aggressive microbe bartonella is the main cause of cat scratch fever.

The pathogen is an intracellular parasite. Preferentially, it invades and infects white blood cells, as well as the endothelial cells, which line the interior membranes of the arteries. Says one investigator, Dr. Ed Breitschwerdt, North Carolina State University professor of veterinary sciences, "The main problem with determining whether bartonella is involved with a particular illness has traditionally been the difficulty of culturing the bacteria from patient samples," again, because it is lodged primarily within cells. There are now reliable means to find it, largely through specialized growth media used to culture the bacteria.

As a result of this new technology the investigators made an astounding finding, which is the fact that humans are literally surrounded by potential sources of this bacteria. Notes Breitschwerdt, "We have found species of bartonella in mammals ranging from mice to sheep to sea otters to dolphins." Of the many species, they discovered some 13 that infect humans. In particular, dogs, cats, cows, and rodents are primary reservoirs, from which the germs are spread to humans by biting insects, not just ticks and fleas but also spiders. Moreover, it is no minor issue, since it is not considered a rare disease. Breitschwerdt also makes this clear, saying that the infection is "one of the most important" of all "untold medical stories."

It is largely "untold" as a result of the means of infection, which is largely through stealth. By the tens of thousands humans are being found infected by bartonella species, the same humans who have a host of chronic illnesses, including Lyme. Other illnesses associated with the infection include migraine headaches, endocarditis or infection of the heart valves, seizures, and rheumatoid arthritis as well as osteoarthritis. These are serious medical syndromes and are commonly listed as 'cause unknown.'

Yet, the symptoms and conditions can often be more diverse, even more destructive, than this. In an article in *North Carolina Health News* the following case was quoted:

> Laura Hopper's tipping point came in 2006, when she was 15 years old. The Raleigh teen lost her peripheral vision. She next began to suffer bouts of joint and muscle pain and numbness in her hands. Then came the headaches, memory loss and hallucination

It was bartonella which was the cause, which she caught most likely from an insect bite. In her case numerous courses of antibiotics were used to clear the infection. Yet, notes Breitschwerdt it is not always this simple:

> "You cannot float humans or horses in enough Doxycycline to kill this bacteria..."

The cat scratch germ or cat scratch-like germ can also cause its own bizarre symptoms and presentation. For instance, it generates purple stretch marks on the buttocks region, thighs, or elsewhere as well as surgical scars, which change from skin tone to a more purple color. When symptoms are all on one side of the body, incredibly, bartonella is often the culprit.

Another indication, says Breitschwerdt, is related to nervous system symptoms. If these symptoms are "out of proportion to the other systemic symptoms of chronic Lyme," then, co-infection by the germ is suspected. The entire nervous system appears to suffer intensively, with symptoms such as agitation, anxiety, insomnia, and even seizures being predominant, leading to other somewhat unexpected Lyme symptoms such as confusion and mental defects that would be expected in cases of encephalitis. Other key symptoms may include gastritis, lower abdominal pain, soreness of the soles, especially upon arising, and tender subcutaneous nodules along the extremities and on occasion, red-colored rashes. Additionally, there may be enlargement of the lymph nodes, especially in the neck and axilla. The neck and/or throat may be sore.

Besides the severe, potentially deadly form there is, commonly, the less extreme type which is rarely fatal even if not treated. Too, a chronic, insidious form can develop. In some instances certain blood parameters may give evidence of bartonella, a co-infector. These parameters include a reduced white count and platelet count as well as elevated liver enzymes.

Oil of wild oregano is invaluable in the treatment of this syndrome. It has the ability to root out the germ from its intracellular hiding spots. Regardless, how can anyone take enough antibiotics to deal with such a broad number of infectious agents: the Lyme bacillus, bartonella, babesia, ehrlichia, tick-borne viruses, mycoplasma, and more? In fact, regarding a number of these they cannot be killed in the least by antibiotic therapy.

In this regard there can be billions upon billions of these pathogens hiding within human cells. For optimal health to be established they must be purged from the body. The oil of wild oregano and the multiple spice complex, as dessicated wild oil capsules, are fully capable of achieving this result.

Babesia

Medicine is nearly always in a highly resistant mode. It blocks any productive change. Seemingly, it has no room for openness. It has fought fiercely against the reality of chronic Lyme. Too, medicine has been slow to realize the scope and danger of co-infections. For instance, when *Babesia microti* was first discovered in humans who had suffered tick bites, it was thought to be the only significant piroplasm affecting them. Now, it is believed that many of the over two dozen known species of piroplasms can be carried by ticks and potentially be transmitted to the human. Despite this, it is almost impossible to determine their existence through any standard testing procedures. There can only be a clinical suspicion based on symptoms.

Rather than bacteria or viruses piroplasms are protozoans. Therefore, by no means will they be eradicated by any of the currently used Lyme treatment regimens. Thus, babesia may readily explain the cause behind those cases that fail to respond to orthodox treatment.

Here is another key to determining this component. It is the fact that co-infection with protozoans results in a more intense level of the acute illness, a greater array of symptoms, and also longer period of time for recovery than Lyme spirochete infection alone. In this regard it has been discovered that spirochete DNA remains in the circulation longer in co-infected subjects than in those experiencing single infection alone. Too, it is held, such a co-infection gives a kind of additional capacity to the spirochete, allowing it to more aggressively attack human joints, heart, and nerves. This is thought to be because babesia infection may impair the native immune defense mechanisms.

It is simple to explain. The immune system is overloaded by the multiplicity of infections. Thus, some of the agents are able to outstrip the immune capacities to prevent their invasion and growth.

It is now known that to some degree Lyme infection consequently implies babesia infestation. It has been published that as many as 66% of Lyme patients show evidence through blood tests of a coincident *Babesia microti* infection.

The range of illness demonstrates its power to corrupt, where it can cause a stealth-like infection but also may cause a severe illness, resulting in hospitalization and even death. What is important here is the fact that subclinical infection is often missed because the symptoms are incorrectly ascribed to Lyme. Too, even in mild cases the infection may later recur, causing severe illness.

Clues to the presence of babesiosis include a more acute initial illness. Patients often recall a high fever and chills at the onset of their Lyme. Over time, they can note night sweats, air hunger, an occasional cough, persistent migraine-like headache, a vague sense of imbalance without true vertigo, encephalopathy, and fatigue. The fulminant presentations are seen in those who are immunosuppressed, especially if asplenic, and in advanced ages. They include high fevers, shaking chills, and hemolysis, which if untreated in such immune-challenged individuals can prove to be fatal.

Mycoplasma

Infections in Lyme disease patients by this agent occur far more commonly than realized. Consisting of a tiny bacteria-like organism, mycoplasma has the propensity to infect both the body fluids as well as the insides of cells. It operates by stealth and largely evades the nervous system. Much of the early work connecting this pathogen to chronic, degenerative disease is attributed to Garth Nicholson, PhD. It was he who determined it to be a common perpetrator of Gulf War illness.

Like Lyme, this infection is a great mimicker. The signs and symptoms of mycoplasma infection are highly variable. As a result, as in Lyme the diagnosis is commonly missed. Some of the primary symptoms and signs of mycoplasma infestation include chronic fatigue, muscular exhaustion, joint pain, intermittent fevers, headaches, nausea, coughing, diarrhea, memory loss, hair loss, light sensitivity, rashes, night sweats, loss of coordination, numbness of the extremities, paralysis, disturbances in digestion, visual disturbances, floaters in the eyes, eye pain, heart failure, problems in urination, and anxiety, among dozens of others. The Nicolson Website at http://www.immed.org lists the full gamut of symptoms, among other information.

Mycoplasma are the typical mutated pathogens well-established to evade immune defenses. So-called pleomorphs, that is organisms which lack a definable cell wall, there is no sound medical treatment, no antibiotic, for curing this infection. There are a number of species of this germ which are pathogenic to humans. The pathogenic species are intracellular parasites; in fact, they must find their way into cells in order to survive. Once there, they evade the immune response and thus become established as permanent residents.

Inside the cells they wreak havoc. They do so by creating free radicals, and these noxious atoms or molecules, then, cause inflammation as well as actual cell destruction. Toxins, including waste products, are released by the mycoplasma into the cells and surrounding fluids. The toxicity can become so overwhelming that the cells begin dying wholesale. When this occurs in the brain and spinal cord, this may result in chronic degenerative disorders such as MS and ALS. In some investigations some 8 of 10 people with ALS were found to have mycoplasma infections, while the weaponized version, *M. fermentans incognitus*, was found in 100% of ALS patients with Gulf War Syndrome.

Nevertheless, one issue is clear, which is the fact that mycoplasma even mimics much of the presentation of Lyme itself. It must always be suspected in tick bite patients who develop chronic fatigue syndrome. Moreover, for those Lyme patients who fail to respond to orthodox therapies the infection by this noxious stealth germ should be considered. Super-strength grade oil of edible wild oregano obliterates this pathogen.

Like Lyme, mycoplasma thrives in cholesterol-rich environments such as the cell membrane, the inside of the cells, and within the brain. Human mycoplasmas have a high need for cholesterol for their growth. According to scientific investigations when activated by stress, these germs become "avid consumers of sterols, including cholesterol."

STARI

While technically not a co-infection this is not the most common tick-borne disaster. Found mainly in the southern, actually, southeastern United States STARI represents an infection by the so-called Lone Star tick. That tick injects a different type of spirochete than seen in Lyme, B. lonestari. The abbreviation stands for Southern-Tick-Associated-Rash-Illness.

The symptoms caused by this infection are similar to those seen in Lyme. This mainly southern tick readily causes a bullseye-like rash. This is associated with the typical Lyme disease symptoms of fatigue, fever, headache, joint pain, muscle paralysis, and muscle pain. In fact, microbiologically, the Lone Star tick spirochete is closely related to *Borrelia burgdorferi*. Like this tick the Lone Star agent can cause neuroborreliosis as well as cardiac spirochete infection. The treatment is the same as that for Lyme disease, with, usually, lesser doses being required to achieve the cure.

Chapter Thirteen

Do's and Don'ts in Fighting Lyme

In Lyme disease it is crucial to avoid stress. Similarly, it is essential to relax as much as possible. Stress aggravates the condition and brings on additional attacks. In fact, it can even cause a relapse in the condition.

Some physicians have found that virtually any kind of stress can have a negative bearing on the condition. This includes the toxic stress from the use of electronic devices, particularly computers and cell phones. In some cases it may be necessary to avoid these entirely, at least until a full-fledged cure is achieved.

Modern electronic devices of the computer age do have a degree of toxicity on the internal organs, especially the brain and nerve centers. In some cases WIFI signals pose great challenges, as the satellite-based signals can irritate the already Lyme-induced trauma to the nerve cells.

Cell phones are highly toxic to the nervous system, particularly the brain. Signals from such phones can cause brain cell death and are associated with the induction of brain cancer. Moreover, cell phone radiation causes damage to the blood-brain barrier, facilitating the invasion by Lyme. In the event of Lyme infestation the use of cell phones should be restricted and/or curtailed.

The Lyme bacillus itself causes disruption of the body's electrochemistry. Like cell phone microwave signals, it causes cell death of both brain and spinal cord cells.

Exercise and movement

Another key means to treat and reverse Lyme disease is movement or exercise. This may be difficult to do when a joint or several joints are seized as a result of inflammation and infestation. Yet, as soon as possible certain types of exercise should be applied.

The most ideal types of exercise for Lyme victims are those which require low amounts of energy and also those which are not major fights against gravity. One such ideal exercise is walking. Once again, this may not be possible in the event of immobility of the key joints for ambulation such as the ankles and knees. Yet, as soon as is possible walking must be instituted. The minimum ideal walk is at least one mile, which should be performed at a relatively brisk speed. Even better is to do two miles or so, that is at least a half hour walk. For optimal results such a walk should be performed daily or at least three times per week.

Yet another type of exercise is at-home calisthenics. These are not just any type of calisthenics but are, rather, a special kind. This special kind is done not standing but instead primarily supine. This takes less energy than exercises done in a standing position and is, therefore, ideal for Lyme disease victims.

These exercises are based on a pumping-like movement. In human physiology all body parts are involved in pumping. So, this is the most natural, physiological exercise known. It is also the most stress-free type of activity. In fact, pumping exercises eliminate stress. This action helps to mobilize the fluids of the body, the arterial blood, the venous blood, the lymph, and the cerebrospinal fluid, so they can re-circulate. The muscle pumping helps pull toxins out of the muscular tissues and joints, cleansing them and, essentially, allowing them to breathe.

Low impact movement is another indoors option. This is through the use of anti-gravity walking machines. With such machines the individual is walking virtually in the air with no contact with the ground. Such exercise is far superior to cardio-style movements such as those done on treadmills and stair walkers.

Bicycling is another option, as is swimming. However, swimming in chlorinated pools is not an option. Chlorine greatly suppresses the immune system and is, in fact, a decided carcinogen.

The low impact, supine exercise system is available as a bound pamphlet, called Pumpercize. To order the Pumpercize bound manual call 1-800-295-3737.

Sunlight and fresh air

What could be more helpful in the reversal of disease than sunlight and fresh air? There can be no doubt about it plenty of sunlight is essential for good health. This does not mean sunbathing in full sun, as this can be immunosuppressive. It just means getting outdoors and being exposed to the natural light, doing so as much as possible. Yet, surely, this must be done while taking the appropriate precautions to avoid exposure to ticks.

Fresh air is also crucial. Oxygen is the ultimate staff of life, acting as the most metabolically crucial substance known. A life indoors can result in a kind of oxygen starvation. Thus, when possible, the Lyme victim must spend time outdoors. This is true even if it means going for a walk and/or sitting on the porch. Oxygen starvation corrupts the function of all the cells and organs in the body. It must be avoided at all costs. The Pumpercize exercise system helps force oxygen into the tissues. It will also stimulate the flow of lymphatic fluid, which is essential in the Lyme disease cure. In good weather these exercises can be done outdoors on a mat.

The main dietary poisons to avoid

No doubt, a person can be readily poisoned by diet. This poisoning suppresses the immune system, making the individual more vulnerable to the noxious effects of the Lyme bacillus while also stalling the healing process. What are these foods and beverages which, if consumed, aggravate the condition? In fact, there are hundreds of such consumables. It is easier to merely list the raw materials used in these foods or drinks; then, these ingredients can be avoided. That avoidance list is as follows:

- refined sugar
- brown sugar

- alcoholic beverages
- corn syrup
- corn starch
- other refined sugars such as refined or adulterated honey, rice syrup, fructose, and grape syrup
- genetically engineered food or food additives
- hydrogenated and partially hydrogenated oils
- refined vegetable oils
- white flour
- white rice

Gluten-containing grains: a major catastrophe

In some instances gluten containing grains prove destructive: to anyone's health. In a person who is gluten intolerant the consumption of gluten-containing grains can cause a vast degree of damage, and this damage may strike virtually any organ in the body. In the case of Lyme disease for those who are intolerant the eating of gluten may greatly impede the recovery from the disease.

Gluten is the protein, a sticky substance, found in common grains such as wheat, rye, barley, and oats. It is also found in certain 'alternative' grains, including kamut and spelt.

Why is this issue so crucial? In the sensitive person gluten becomes a cause of pathology. It actually has the capacity to destroy tissues, particularly the lining of the gut. Here, it causes direct toxicity to the most critical component of the intestinal system, which is the absorptive surface organ known as the intestinal villi. The villi, actually, villous membrane, is the region where food, once digested, is absorbed.

Represented by tiny invaginations the ultimate breadth of the villous membrane system is vast. If all these little tips were flattened out, it would amount to, incredibly, the same breadth of surface area as a tennis court.

It's a delicate system. Sticky gluten causes a noxious reaction leading to the denuding, that is obliteration, of the absorptive surface. This may reduce the assimilation of nutrients by some 95%.

It is not just the issue of digestive status that is corrupted. The immune system also is severely compromised as a result of such damage. The intestinal villi play a major role in a healthy immune system of the gut but also the rest of the body. They are an anatomic cohort to the immune organ of the gut, known as the Peyer's Patches. These patches are, essentially, embedded lymphatic nodules within the small intestinal wall. For nourishment they are reliant on healthy intestinal villi. When the villi are destroyed, simultaneously, so are the Peyer's Patches. Some 60% of the mass of lymph tissue in the body consists of these patchy lymphatic nodules. The patchy tissue is responsible for the production of not only lymphocytes but also key immune proteins known as immunoglobulins.

Regarding the gut one of these immunoglobulins is particularly important. Known as secretory IgA this immune protein is essential for optimal health of the intestinal canal through its entirety. Secretary IgA is needed by the gut to bind any noxious agent, whether allergic-causing protein or germ. This binding is necessary in order to neutralize the toxin or pathogen in order for it to be destroyed. The consumption of gluten-containing grains and milk protein, that is casein, causes a reduction in the levels of this essential antibody complex. In some cases because of such food reactions the levels of secretory IgA are virtually obliterated from the body. Put simply, both casein and gluten cause the consumption of these immunologically active compounds.

Thus, it is essential for potentially gluten-sensitive people to eliminate all such grains from the diet. Of note, this diet relies heavily on rice-based foods, which are an ideal alternative for gluten-rich grain-based foods. Too, for other sources of starch potatoes and sweet potatoes are recommended alternatives. For the gluten intolerant person if gluten-containing foods are vigorously avoided, gradually, the chronic infection state generally improves.

Are natural foods toxic?

With the revelation of the toxicity of gluten-containing grains it becomes clear that developing a Lyme disease cure diet is not so easy. In this regard could other whole, natural foods be an issue? Could they, too, aggravate the disease? In fact, this is surely true in some instances. Too, it must be kept in mind that certain foods can induce inflammation in the body. For instance, joint swelling and even arthritis is associated with the consumption of specific foods, including milk products, shrimp, grains, and in some cases plants of the nightshade family such as tomatoes and eggplant. Surely, any food which might cause inflammation of the joints should be avoided in severe Lyme cases. For instance, the consumption of beans, lentils, and seafood can bring on a gout attack, as can the intake of organ meats and red meat.

What are these provocative foods? Many foods are well established for their allergy-causing potential as well as their capacity to induce inflammation in the body. They are mainly foods of the milk and grain category, although in some individuals eggs are a major toxin. Regarding milk, it is cow's milk and cow's milk products that are primarily at issue. With grains, wheat is the major Lyme antagonist, although all the gluten-containing grains may well be necessary to avoid. It is these grains, along with cow's milk products, which must be primarily avoided in order to prevent aggravation or recurrence of the disease. Thus, for people with allergic or gluten sensitivity issues the key foods, then, to avoid in order to reverse Lyme disease are as follows:

- wheat
- rye
- gluten-containing oats (gluten-free oats are now available and can be used as an alternative)
- barley
- commercial cow's milk as well as cow's milk yogurt and cheese
- cow's milk butter

> Note: in some cases organic cow's milk yogurt, full-fat, may well be tolerated. It may be necessary to experiment with it in order to determine if it is non-reactive. Even so, in countless millions of people the consumption of such foods leads to a suppression of the immune system, disruption of digestion, and as mentioned previously in the case of gluten-containing grains actual destruction of the digestive surfaces. With such a degree of sensitivity, how can a person survive, let alone thrive?

For some people milk protein, casein, can be equally destructive, although the consequences are different. Casein can prove highly damaging to the delicate walls of the colon. This surely leads to irritable bowel and in extreme cases ulcerative colitis. There is no reason to endure such toxicity when the solution is so simple. For those who are vulnerable all that is necessary is to eliminate such foods and their derivatives.

Will this prove difficult? It would be if a person could only rely on processed food. With a true whole food diet the elimination of gluten-containing grains and cow's milk products is actually a minor issue. There are hundreds of other foods to select from. Moreover, regarding starch there is always brown rice, potatoes, and sweet potatoes. In the case of milk products sheep's and/or goat's milk foods are now commonly available. In some areas it is even possible to procure buffalo milk-based foods.

On this diet gluten-containing grains and their derivatives, as well as cow's milk-based foods, are eliminated. The exception is organic cow's milk butter, which may be tolerated by those with modest milk sensitivities. In any menu or recipe calling for butter it can be substituted with goat's milk butter, extra virgin olive oil, coconut oil, red palm oil, and/or crude cold-pressed pumpkinseed oil.

In addition, the consumption of certain excessively sweet foods, such as sweet potatoes, pears, and apples, should be limited, and it is essential not to go overboard on the consumption of white potatoes. Regarding apples and pears, if organic, the skins can be eaten. Raisins and prunes should also be eaten only in limited amounts, while regarding grapes, plain table grapes are too sweet. The more tart organic red and purple grapes are preferable. Ideally, look for grapes which still contain the seed, as these are closer to the original cultivars than the highly hybridized seedless grapes. The reason that this diet is not excessively strict on fresh grapes is that they are highly cleansing to the intestinal tract and kidneys.

Too, raw, wild honey has significant cleansing powers. It is also medicinal, containing natural antiseptics and antibiotics, including formic acid and a special antibiotic unique to raw honey alone. The two top medicinal honeys to consume are manuka and wild oregano honey. Yet, in people with candida overload even honey must often be restricted, that is until the fungus infestation is reversed. In some cases the natural sugars allowed on this diet can be better tolerated if a person consumes the wild oregano oil aggressively on a daily basis, since this helps obliterate any candida or other yeasts circulating in the blood or lodged into the gut.

Even non-nutritive sweeteners, such as stevia and sorbitol, may cause an aggravation in the Lyme condition. Stick to the high-protein, high-fat foods as the primary nutrition source. This is backed up with fruit and vegetables. This is the most ideal anti-Lyme diet conceivable, which through the low carbohydrate nature of the diet blocks the growth of carbohydrate-rich, sticky biofilms.

Do alcohol and Lyme mix?

For Lyme disease alcohol, too, is a no-no. For complete recovery to occur its consumption should be strictly curtailed. That includes fermented beverages such as wine and beer. Alcohol is a decided metabolic poison. It directly intoxicates the white blood cells, causing their destruction. It also has a noxious effect on the bone marrow, blocking the production of new white blood cells. Too, it can directly cause cell death of red blood cells.

Its toxic effects on the digestive system are well established. A major cause of stomach ulcers it has a strong action against the gastric lining. One major condition that it causes is gastric atrophy, that is death of the stomach's cell lining. This leads to a wide range of digestive and metabolic disorders. Ultimately, it leads to gastric cancer. Alcohol is also a key cause of ulcers of both the stomach and duodenum.

Then, too, its major arena of toxicity is the liver. It is this organ which must deal with the brunt of this poison's metabolic actions. When this chemical is consumed, it is broken down to even more poisonous compounds, including acetaldehyde and formaldehyde. These substances are deliberate cellular poisons. The consequence is cell death of liver cells and, ultimately, cirrhosis of this organ.

There is another key issue regarding its extreme toxicity. As mentioned previously alcohol is highly toxic to the brain, including the blood-brain barrier. Regarding that barrier it greatly corrupts it, causing it to become excessively weak and thin. In particular, studies have shown that alcohol directly poisons the cell components of this barrier, the lining cells, the endothelial cells, and the neurological ones, the astrocytes. The purpose of the blood brain barrier is to protect this organ from toxic substances but also to guard it from infection. Furthermore, alcohol itself intoxicates the immune system, increasing the vulnerability to bacterial infections. Simultaneously, it causes great damage to the key cells of the brain such as the astrocytes. It is, importantly, these cells which are essential for aiding in the repair of damaged brain cells. It has already been determined that the Lyme spirochete can directly penetrate that barrier. Alcohol corrupts the precise mechanism needed for brain cell regeneration in the event of neuroborreliosis.

Through its toxic actions on a wide range of organs alcohol damages the tissues to such a degree that the regular consumption of alcoholic beverages can cause a relapse in the disease. Therefore, in the case of Lyme disease or the co-infections avoid this poison like the plague.

So, what is a person to consume for pleasure if the alcoholic beverages, wheat products, and refined sugar are taken away? Wild, raw honey can be used on this diet. So can certain types of fruit juice. Organic carrot juice can also be consumed, and this is delicious. This juice has potent healing properties. Curiously, it is a natural antiseptic. These sweet foods/beverages will not impair the Lyme disease recovery. Pure organic grape juice is allowed, as it is highly cleansing on the body. In particular, it aids in the cleansing and rebuilding of the arteries as well as the intestinal canal. Only purple or red grape juice should be consumed.

Excessively sweet fruit juice should be avoided, however, such as apple juice and processed orange juice. In contrast, freshly squeezed apple and orange juice are acceptable, as are freshly squeezed pear, pineapple, and papaya juice.

Organic carrot juice: tissue healing agent

Is carrot juice a part of the Lyme cure? It sure is an essential component of any cancer reversal plan. This is largely a result of the cleansing properties of this juice. It is also related to its germicidal powers. It may well be the most antiseptic of all vegetables. In this regard what stays intact longer, with or without refrigeration, than carrots? Carrots are an excellent source of trace minerals, much needed for reviving stressed or diseased cells. It is also a good source of vitamin B. The nutrients in carrot juice are readily digested and absorbed into the body. Thus, there is heavy use of raw organic carrot juice on this diet, since its consumption will speed the recovery and the cure.

One of the reasons for its powers relates to its content of trace minerals. The primary minerals found in the juice are calcium, phosphorous, potassium, and sodium. The sodium content is significant, as this helps bolster adrenal function. Vitamins C, D, E, K, thiamine, and pyridoxine are also found in significant amounts. The tops are a rich source of potassium and that rather rare nutrient, vitamin K. These, too, can be juiced and added to the root juice. Because of its dense supply of nutrients it is not only rejuvenating for the body but is also highly cleansing and, in fact, exceedingly invigorating, especially for those suffering from chronic disease.

GMOs – Lyme provocateurs?

GMO-tainted foods are highly destructive to the human body. In particular, they are exceedingly noxious in their actions on the immune system. Thus, in the case of Lyme disease their consumption must be strictly avoided. The primary GMO-infested foods are as follows:

- corn
- soy
- canola
- cottonseed oil and meal
- beet sugar
- Hawaiian papayas
- yellow crooked neck squash

> Note: when any such foods and/or their derivatives are found on labels, such foods must be absolutely avoided. The derivatives are many. These derivatives include:

- corn syrup
- corn starch
- dextrin
- dextrose
- citric acid
- ascorbic acid
- tocopherol
- alpha tocopherol
- corn oil
- soybean oil
- vegetable oil
- hydrogenated vegetable oil
- partially hydrogenated vegetable oil
- cottonseed oil
- canola oil
- fructose
- glucose
- invert syrup
- glucose syrup

For anyone with tick-based infections it is crucial to avoid the consumption of GMOs at all costs. The noxious foods and food derivatives are highly immunosuppressive. It would be no easy task to prevail in the battle against Lyme disease if such foods are routinely consumed. The destruction they wreak is vast. French studies confirm that GMOs are deliberate carcinogens and that they cause in animals monstrous-sized tumors. The body needs the vital energy derived from whole, natural foods.

Therefore, the diet should consist of farm-fresh foods and organic foods as much as possible. Moreover, by no means should any GMO-tainted foods be consumed on this diet.

Fish and Fukushima

Radiation from the detonations of the Fukushima nuclear plants is a real issue in respect to a healthy diet. The majority of this radiation has dumped or fallen directly into the ocean, primarly the Pacific Ocean, the Bering Sea, and the northern Pacific Ocean. As a consequence the sea creatures in these seas are becoming radioactive. This is a serious issue. The overconsumption of Pacific Ocean-source fish may significantly increase the risks for certain diseases, notably diseases of the thyroid, including nodule formation and thyroid cancer, as well as leukemia, lymphoma, sarcoma, bone cancer, among others. For this reason the consumption of fish from the Pacific ocean must be limited or curtailed.

Chapter Fourteen

Nutrients Against Lyme

There are a number of key nutrients that aid in the battle against Lyme disease and the various co-infection agents. These are nutrients which are rather rare in the food supply and may be regarded as substances found primarily in foods of high nutrient density. Some of these nutrients are known by the distinction, Factor X as coined by Weston Price, DOS. These absolutely key nutrients are vitamin C, the B complex, vitamin A, vitamin D, and vitamin K. Factor X mainly applies to the fat soluble ones, A, D, and K.

There are a litany of other crucial nutrients such as the trace minerals and vitamin E. The focus, though, will be on the ones which act directly and aggressively in the reversal of the Lyme pathology.

Vitamin A: anti-Lyme nutrient and more

This fat soluble vitamin is essential for strong immune

defenses. Vitamin A is needed for the production of key immune proteins known as antibodies. In particular, the synthesis of a highly potent antibody, secretory IgA, is dependent upon adequate vitamin A status. There is some data demonstrating the need for this key substance in the battle against Lyme. In an animal study on mice it was determined that vitamin A deficiency increases the vulnerability for developing Lyme-related inflammation. In fact, vitamin A is a kind of natural cortisone-like agent.

Only natural-source vitamin A can be depended upon for this positive effect. Top food sources include beef or calf's liver, or lamb liver (only organic sources must be used), fish liver oils, fish oils extracted from fish heads, roe, fatty fish, and egg yolk. As it can be seen the food sources of this vitamin are limited. The top natural supplemental source is fatty salmon oil from wild sockeye salmon. This oil is made from the heads of this fish through steam extraction. It is the only entirely natural source fish oil available that is a dense source of naturally occurring vitamin A. For Lyme disease a minimum of 2000 IUs of natural-based vitamin A should be consumed. Fatty steam extracted salmon oil is available as an 8-ounce bottle or in 1000 mg capsules. This is a case where more is usually better, as the 'side-effect' is improved circulation and a reduction of the development of coronary artery disease. The fatty salmon oil has also been noted to reduce the intensity of menopausal symptoms, likely a result of its dense supplies of vitamin A. That vitamin is needed for the reduction of inflammation in the ovaries as well as for the ovarian synthesis of estrogen, progesterone, and other steroidal hormones.

The deficiency is crucial in a number of respects. A lack of it makes the tissues highly vulnerable to infection, in particular, on the skin, within the kidneys, within the gut, and in the bloodstream. These are areas readily traumatized by the Lyme bacillus. Too, the lymphatic organs themselves are dependent upon vitamin A for regeneration. What this means is that for a person who is deficient in this key immune-supporting nutrient the contraction of Lyme after a tick bite is likely, that is compared to a person who has healthy vitamin A nutrition.

It has to do with the capacity of the immune response and how it is compromised in the deficiency. It has been demonstrated that in order to clear the Lyme bacillus a strong immune system is required, specifically the naturally existing macrophage system, along with the antibody-mediated one, where these anti-germ proteins are produced specifically against the Lyme spirochete. Both the production of macrophages and antibodies is dependent upon adequate levels of vitamin A. Thus, to fully eradicate the spirochetal infection plentiful amounts of the vitamin must be ingested. For Lyme disease cases the intake of naturally vitamin A-rich fatty salmon oil is a must.

B complex

Like vitamin A, the B vitamins are essential for immune health as well as overall energy and strength. Their deficiency greatly weakens the body. Gross deficiency leads to muscular weakness, fatigue, irritability, anxiety, depression, digestive disturbances, blood sugar disorders, overall weakness, poor appetite, heart palpitations, a sensation of being cold, aches and pains, bloating, numbness, tingling, burning of the tongue, burning or pain in the heels of the feet, headaches, swelling, including edema of the legs and feet, and memory loss, among others. Curiously, many of these symptoms are also seen in Lyme disease. Therefore, it is crucial in the fight against this condition to maintain good B vitamin nutrition in the body. The recipes in this book will help that. So will the consumption of the all-natural whole food B complex powder described herein.

In contrast, the consumption of the standard B complex sources, pressed pills and capsules, will not resolve the deficit. In fact, these may aggravate it, since the B vitamins in such sources are synthetic or semi-synthetic. It is now known that such artificial vitamins upon absorption into the body cause considerable damage, including blocking the absorption of naturally occurring B vitamins, the ones found in food and food concentrates. Plus, such synthetic vitamins contain a number of dangerous toxins which disrupt the health of people who are chronically ill. These toxins are coal tar and petrochemical derivatives. Both coal tar and gasoline-like molecules are used as the basis upon which many vitamins are produced. Other toxins used in the production of vitamins include refined vegetable oils, sewage waste, cattle brains, and GMO corn derivatives.

In Lyme the nervous system is struck severely. It is the B complex that is needed to regenerate this system. Thus, follow the food plan in this book. Consume foods rich in naturally occurring B vitamins. Also, regularly take the whole food B complex supplement recommended, here. Top food sources of the B complex include the following:

rice bran
organic liver
torula yeast
brewer's yeast
royal jelly
brown rice
sunflower seeds

almonds
spinach
kale
dark green lettuce
dandelion greens
cheese
wild rice
wheat germ
oat bran
eggs
wild salmon
sardines
wild tuna (a challenge, since much of this is overloaded with mercury and tainted by Fukushima radiation)
wild chaga
wild mushrooms
freshly squeezed orange juice

Of note, regarding many of these foods they are rarely consumed by the average individual. Therefore, surely, even among people living in Western countries gross deficiency is common. People think they have this covered by taking pressed pills and other sources of the B complex. It is not resolved from this. They must replenish low and declining reservoirs from the vitamins of nature. For Lyme disease victims an intake of foods rich in the B complex, as well as food based B vitamin supplements, is essential for the cure.

Vitamin C

If there was a focus for Lyme disease and co-infection conditions regarding vitamin intake, it would be vitamins A, the B complex, vitamin D, and vitamin C. Regarding the latter this is obviously essential for immune function as well as for the fight against inflammation.

This is one of the most crucial vitamins in the battle against Lyme disease. It is a key factor for vital life, and its deficiency greatly weakens the body. Most obviously, a deficiency of vitamin C leads to the weakening of blood vessel walls, leading to various kinds of hemorrhaging or vulnerability to such hemorrhaging. In this regard it must be recognized that the vitamin is required for the production of intracellular cement, essentially, cellular glue.

With spirochete infection the strength and health of that glue is crucial. A strong body structure based upon plentiful intake of vitamin C is a massive defense against Lyme invasion. Notes Cooper in *Nutrition in Health and Disease* the vitamin has a "highly significant role in the formation and maintenance of...intracellular cement-like substance..." Intracellular cement—what can be more crucial than that?

A deficiency of vitamin C leads to gross damage of the various tissues dependent upon such cement, the skin, ligaments, tendons, muscles, joints, bones, gums, teeth, and even the internal organs themselves. Normal healing of wounds is also dependent upon it, as is the normal, vital function of the immune system. Furthermore, it is poorly stored in the body, a fact which is thoroughly established. Notes Cooper: any excess of vitamin C is 'promptly' excreted by the body, demonstrating the "limited powers" within the body for the storage of the nutrient.

Therefore, it is crucial to consume vitamin C on a regular basis. Yet, such consumption is particularly indicated in any infection, whether acute or chronic. Infection causes the rapid consumption of this nutrient, while fevers cause it to be rapidly consumed as well as aggressively excreted. Vitamin C is readily destroyed by cooking. Therefore, a diet based largely on cooked food is usually significantly deficient. The top food and/or supplemental sources of this vitamin are relatively few, as follows, largely in order from highest density to lowest:

camu camu
acerola cherry
rose hips
oranges
orange juice (freshly squeezed)
lemons and lemon juice
limes and lime juice
organic liver
strawberries
grapefruit
broccoli
turnip greens
cantaloupe
green pepper
red sweet pepper
cauliflower
Brussels sprouts
raspberries
tomato juice (freshly squeezed)
tomatoes, raw
potato, baked

If a person is not consuming such dense food sources on a daily or every-other-day basis, such a one is grossly deficient in the vitamin. Vitamin C supplements don't correct this, because they are made from dead material: mere GMO-tainted, solvent-treated corn. Only vitamin C supplements made from wild plants contain purely natural vitamin C. All other supplements claiming to be natural sources of the vitamin are fraudulent.

The bone builders, vitamins D & K

The bone-building vitamins, D and K, are essential nutrients in the Lyme defense plan. The Lyme spirochete causes great corruption in the bone and joint system. It breaks this system down. Thus, in order to defeat this disease process powerful bone-repairing and building nutrients are essential. Top food sources of vitamin D include cod liver oil, wild sockeye salmon oil, fish liver, lamb's liver, calf's liver, cow's liver, kidney, wild salmon, fish roe, sardines, and egg yolk. The best natural whole-food source of vitamin D available is PolarPower fatty salmon oil, available as capsules or in an 8-ounce bottle. Sources of vitamin K include fish liver, burbot liver, burbot liver oil (OmegaADK), lambs or cow's liver, dandelion greens, kale, romaine lettuce, bibb lettuce, red leaf lettuce, broccoli, cabbage, spinach, asparagus, and fermented soy foods.

Regarding the bones there is a special supplement available for building them. Based on the latest research this supplement consists of a potent bone-building form of calcium, raw bone from grass-fed New Zealand cattle. The active ingredient of this bone complex is known as hydroxyapatite. This substance is combined with wild spices known to enhance bone formation, notably wild rosemary, oregano, and sage. This bone-activating supplement is available as 550 mg capsules and also as a potent rubbing oil. Combined with natural sources of vitamin D and vitamin K, it is ideal for assisting the body in the re-mineralization of bone.

The most powerful source of all of these bone strengthening vitamins is wild burbot oil. This oil is derived from the livers of a far northern fish also known as the mariah.The mariah is essentially a type of freshwater cod. This species of fish is an exceptionally dense source of fat soluble vitamins. It is one of the rare natural sources of bone building vitamin K.

Upon one of my relapses with Lyme there was considerable damage to the left knee. That damage was slow in healing. The addition of wild burbot oil not as an extract oil but rather, as a raw, whole liver complex, along with the use of oil of oregano and deep-eezing oil as rubbing oils, dramatically increased the rate of healing of the knee. The flexibility of the knee joint was increased significantly through the intake of this raw liver complex, known as Omega-ADK.

It must be emphasized that the key to its powers is its rawness. Omega-ADK is the only raw, freshwater vitamin-rich fish liver oil available. Clearly, then, raw, unheated vitamins are more potent than cooked/heat treated varieties. Especially with fat soluble vitamins heat causes kinking, that is corruption, of the molecular structure. In the wild animals devour the flesh and organs of freshwater cod. No wonder; they need it for their sustenance and strength. Omega-ADK is only available through special order through the Website, www.cassingram.com. It's handmade in small batches and so is quite rare. A few high quality health food stores may carry it in the supplement refrigeration section.

Cholesterol: a key Lyme fighting nutrient

Can anyone fathom it? The yellow wax cholesterol is absolutely an essential nutrient, particularly in Lyme disease.

This is because it is tissue cholesterol that is one of the front-line defenses against spirochete attack. The germ attacks the membranes of the cells, and these membranes are made largely from this lipid. Furthermore, it would appear a number of the infectious agents occurring in tick bite diseases, notably borrelia and mycoplasma, actually consume the cholesterol in the body as food. The diet in this book is super-rich in animal-source cholesterol. It is also high in the plant form of this substance, known as plant sterols. The ideal supplemental source of plant sterols is wild chaga, especially raw forms, like raw chaga sublingual drops. Raw Austrian-source pumpkinseed oil is yet another excellent source, as is black seed oil. Excellent food sources include red palm oil, wild herbs, and sunflower seeds as well as sunflower seed butter and also nuts, along with nut butter, in general.

Chapter Fifteen

Recipes and Menus

Two Weeks of Eating Right

Day One

Breakfast
two or three eggs over easy
BetaPalmed Gluten Free Toast*
glass freshly squeezed organic carrot juice or grapefruit juice

Snack
pistachio nuts
glass V-8 juice

Lunch
Organic Carrot 'n Pea Vegetable Patties*
tossed salad with feta cheese; extra virgin olive oil, black seed oil, and vinegar
herbal tea or spring water

Snack
veggie sticks plus slices of goat's cheese
slices organic turkey or beef
mineral water

Dinner
Organic Calf's Liver with Sage*
tossed salad
bowl of wild berries topped with raw honey and walnuts
herb tea

Day Two

Breakfast
bowl organic full fat cottage cheese with raw berries of your choice
oat bran cereal topped with butter and raw honey
wild chaga tea (Chag-o-Charge or ChagaBlack)

Snack
salted roasted almonds and V-8 juice
fresh vegetable juice with fresh lemon and a hint of sea salt

Lunch
Fresh Wild Rice Organic Chicken Soup*
tossed salad of your choice
chunks of melon
spring water

Snack
ChagaChunks
wild tamarack bark (larch bark) or birch bark tea

Dinner
Simple Clay Pot Baked Organic Chicken*
romaine lettuce salad
wedges avocado and grapefruit
mineral water

Day Three

Breakfast
2 boiled organic eggs
bowl oat bran cereal topped with cinnamon, almond milk, and raw honey

Snack
grapefruit slices and chunks of melon, salted
salted, roasted nuts of your choice
tomato juice or mineral water

Lunch
organic hamburger, any style, on gluten-free bread
Tomato-Cucumber Salad*
glass fresh-extracted organic carrot juice

Snack
veggie sticks
nut butter as a dip or spread

Dinner
Turkey Meatloaf*
Popeye Salad*
grapefruit slices
mineral water or chaga tea

Day Four

Breakfast
Spinach and Feta Cheese Salad*
one or two pieces gluten-free toast, well buttered
glass grapefruit or pomegranate juice

Snack
ChagaChunks
cup wild chaga tea (Chag-o-Charge or ChagaDunkers)

Lunch
Greenwich Roll-Ups*
fresh vegetable juice of your choice with a bit of sea salt

Snack
nuts of your choice
mineral water

Dinner
Organic Calf's Liver with Sage*
tossed salad
Pineapple and Melon Cocktail*
wild chaga and dandelion tea (ChagaBrew)

Day Five

Breakfast
bowl organic goat's or sheep's yogurt with berries
oat bran cereal topped with butter and raw honey
glass grapefruit or freshly squeezed orange juice

Snack
few pieces of feta cheese
veggie sticks
mineral water

Lunch
roast beef sandwich on gluten-free bread or bun; mustard as a dressing
tossed green salad; extra virgin olive oil and vinegar
glass mineral or chlorine-free water

Snack
glass organic carrot juice
salted roasted almonds

Dinner
Fresh Wild Rice Organic Chicken Soup*

tossed salad of any kind
cup ChagaBlack tea or ChagaDunkers tea

Day Six

Breakfast
bowl of gluten-free cereal(s) of choice, topped with raw, organic sunflower seeds and raisins
unsweetened hemp or almond milk
raw honey (optional for adding to the cereal, freshly ground for easier digestion)
wedge honeydew or cantaloupe
cup wild chaga tea (ChagaDunkers)

> Note: for this breakfast in order to stabilize the blood sugar add a goodly amount of sunflower seeds to the cereal

Snack
slices of organic beef or bison with red sweet peppers
fresh-squeezed carrot juice

Lunch
baked whitefish (ideally, real wild whitefish but select whatever is available, like haddock, cod, or other)
tossed salad
mineral water

Snack
greek olives
sliced tomatoes
mineral water with lemon

Dinner
Natural Beef Meat loaf*
Rich Romaine and Feta Cheese Salad*
White Radish Soup*
Pomegranate Bubbly Surprise*

Day Seven

Breakfast
sardines or kippers over a bed of sliced tomatoes and lettuce
two pieces gluten-free toast, well buttered
wild chaga tea

Snack
left-over meatloaf or other cold meat
glass grapefruit and papaya juice (mixed 50/50)

Lunch
organic or grass-fed hamburger smothered with onions and mushrooms
mustard as a relish
tossed salad dressed with extra virgin olive oil and vinegar
mineral water

Snack
cherry tomatoes and salt
chunks of cheese
mineral water

Dinner
Organic Carrot 'n Pea Vegetable Patties*
Organic Minty Cantaloupe Soup*
a bit of sliced roast turkey, if desired, or slices of eggs
chaga or wild dandelion root tea (both are available as HealthHunter ChagaBrew)

Week Two

Day One

Breakfast
two or three eggs over easy
sliced tomatoes and onions
wedge cantaloupe
herbal tea

Snack
small squares feta cheese
english walnuts
herbal tea or fresh vegetable juice

Lunch
bison burger (or, if unavailable, grass-fed beef burger)
sliced onions and tomatoes
mustard
spring water

Snack
salted pistachios
glass grapefruit juice

Dinner
baked wild fish (ideally, not from the Pacific Ocean due to issues of Fukushima radiation contamination)
steamed broccoli and/or Brussels sprouts—olive oil or butter
bowl mixed fruit topped with natural whipping cream and honey, if desired
chaga tea (as Chaga Dunkers or Chag-o-Charge Tea)

Day Two

Breakfast
healthy gluten-free cereal with almond or hemp milk, topped with walnuts and berries
wedge watermelon
wild chaga tea

Snack
greek olives and slices of avocado
tomato juice with lemon

Lunch
Special Chopped Sardine Salad*
boiled egg

grapefruit slices
mineral water or herbal tea

Snack
sliced turkey meat or left-over meat loaf
glass organic purple or red grape juice

Dinner
glass of fresh-extracted organic carrot juice
Diced Fruit 'n Nut Yogurt Iced Surprise*

Day Three

Breakfast
Italian Omelet*
wedge cantaloupe or honeydew
cup wild chaga tea

Snack
wild pecans and/or walnuts
dried apricots

Lunch
Beef Bacon Flavored Brussel Sprouts*
Garden Soup*
bowl of berries

Snack
sliced organic turkey or chicken meat
slices of red sweet pepper

Dinner

Pureed Fish Creamy Soup*
Traditional Greek Salad*
glass tomato juice with lemon and sea salt

Day Four

Breakfast
three egg omelet
sliced tomatoes
wedge cantaloupe or honeydew
cup wild chaga tea (as ChagaDunkers or Chag-o-Charge tea)

Snack
macadamia or pistachio nuts
glass grapefruit juice

Lunch
Double-Decker King Oscar Sardine Sandwich*
melon wedges
mineral water

Snack
red sweet pepper slices and slices of goat's cheese
half roasted organic or free range chicken

Dinner
Curried Organic Lamb*
Extra-Rich Squash Soup*
tossed salad
chaga tea

Day Five

Breakfast
Raw Egg Almond Milk Carob Shake*
red sweet pepper slices with slices goat's cheese; drizzle with
Mediterranean pomegranate syrup

Snack
handful mixed, salted nuts
glass fresh-extracted organic carrot juice

Lunch
salad with wild salmon; extra virgin olive oil and vinegar dressing
Mashed Potato Puffs*
herbal tea

Snack
turkey or alpaca sticks
glass grapefruit juice

Dinner
Organic Steak and Tomato Casserole*
Fruit Salad with Coconut-Lime Dressing*
glass organic carrot juice*

Day Six

Breakfast
oat bran cereal with added wild pecan or walnut chunks, cinnamon, and raw honey
organic strawberries

Snack
cheese slices and veggie sticks
cup ChagaBlack tea

Lunch
glass fresh-extracted organic carrot juice
Herb-Buttered Parsnip Strips*
Organic Liver and Dandelion Salad*
herbal tea

Snack
turkey jerkey or alpaca jerkey sticks
sliced veggies
mineral water

Dinner
steak or lamb of any kind cooked in red palm oil
fried onions in the palm oil
tossed salad dressed with extra virgin olive oil, lemon, and vinegar
Roasted Whole Head Cauliflower*

Day Seven

Breakfast
turkey or beef sausages (or nitrate-free hot dogs)
raw sliced onions
one or two eggs over easy or poached
half grapefruit or cantaloupe wedges
cup chaga tea (either as ChagaDunkers or Chag-o-Charge Wild Forest Tea)

Snack
mixed salted nuts
mineral water or tomato juice

Lunch
tossed salad topped with sardines or herring
bunch of organic or chemical-free purple or red grapes
handful of walnuts
mineral or spring water

Snack
celery and carrot sticks, salted
slices goat's or sheep's cheese

Dinner
organic steak smothered with onions and mushrooms
roasted new potatoes
steamed green or yellow wax beans, well buttered
Fruit Salad with Coconut Lime Dressing*
glass grapefruit juice

RECIPES: ENTREES

Simple Baked Clay Pot Organic Chicken

Oil of wild oregano greatly tenderizes poultry. It will, though, give it a healthy oregano taste, but this is such a novel treatment, because the meat becomes so tender that it literally falls off the bone. For this purpose only use the P73 type, as this is the wild food-grade oregano, which offers to the poultry a rich flavor.

½ pound organic chicken parts or more (as much as will fit in the clay pot)
8 carrots, cleaned, ends removed, cut in two-inch chunks
2 or more white potatoes, cleaned and cut into pieces (leave skin on)
2 large onions, chopped in eighths
¼ stick organic butter
one or two T. extra virgin olive oil
red sour grape powder (if available)
mediterranean pomegranate syrup (optional; gives a sweet and sour element)
miscellaneous spices of your choice

Preheat oven to 350 degrees. Wash chicken parts well; rub with wild oregano oil. Place as much as possible in the clay pot, leaving room for the potatoes, onions, and carrots. Add carrots, onions, and potatoes, then add butter and sprinkle with extra virgin olive oil, then add red sour grape, sea salt, and spices; drizzle with pomegranate syrup. Place covered in clay pot in the oven; cook for 1 1/2 hours then test to see if it is tender. Cook until the meat is done (when you test it with a fork, it's tender through and through).

Sautéed Spinach, Mediterranean-Style with Feta Cheese and Olives

1 T. extra virgin olive oil
2 T. golden raisins
1 T. pine nuts
2 cloves garlic, minced

2 T. finely minced organic red sweet peppers
1 10-ounce bag fresh, organic spinach, tough stems removed
1 T. balsamic vinegar
½ tsp. sea salt
1 T. shaved Parmesan cheese
freshly ground pepper to taste

In a large skillet or dutch oven heat oil over medium-high heat. Add raisins, pine nuts and garlic; cook, stirring until fragrant, about 3 minutes. Add spinach and red sweet peppers and cook, stirring until just wilted, about 2 minutes. Remove from heat; stir in vinegar and salt. Serve immediately, sprinkled with Parmesan and pepper.

Natural Beef Stroganoff with Wild Mushrooms

Typically, with Beef Stroganoff alcohol is used, either as beer or cognac. Since alcohol is often noxious for Lyme patients, this is avoided. Instead, a combination of brewer's yeast and honey is used to gain the alcohol, that is yeasty flavoring.

12 oz. organic beef fillet or sandwich steak
3 T. organic butter
1 yellow onion, minced
¼ cup mushrooms
1 T. extra virgin olive oil
1 cup heavy cream
1 T. brewer's yeast
1 T. raw honey
sea salt
freshly ground black pepper

Chop beef into chunks. Brown them slowly in extra virgin olive oil. Add onions and butter and cook until done or clear. Add mushrooms; cook covered until steak is tender. Add heavy cream, brewer's yeast, and honey, and a dash of sea salt and pepper. Serve as is or over a bed of wild and brown rice or brown rice noodles.

Lamb's Kidneys and Scrambled Eggs

2 organic lamb's kidneys
4 organic eggs
2 oz. organic butter
contents 4 OregaMax capsules
HerbSorb or Herbamere
curry powder
1 T. freshly squeezed lemon juice
sea salt
pepper
red palm oil
4 pieces gluten-free bread

Cut kidneys into small pieces, season well. Heat butter, and cook for about 8 minutes, adding a T. of water to prevent sticking, if necessary. Add lemon juice. Beat and season eggs lightly. Add to kidney, and continue cooking until firm. Set aside, covered. In a skillet heat red palm oil (or butter, if this is not available). Cook bread until firm or somewhat stiff. Serve kidneys over fried bread.

Moroccan Harissa Lamb

1 T. harissa (see Americanwildfoods.com), plus extra to serve
1¾ lbs. lamb fillets, trimmed
¼ cup extra virgin olive oil
2 carrots, thinly sliced
1 medium red onion, thinly sliced
12 black Greek olives, seeds removed
1 14 oz. can chickpeas, drained
1 tsp. ground ginger
1 tsp. ground cumin
handful of coriander leaves
1 T. finely grated lemon zest, plus 1 T. lemon juice
1 T. raw honey
4 T. full fat yogurt

Spread the harissa over the lamb to coat. Heat 1 T. oil in a fry pan over medium-high heat and cook the lamb, turning, for 2-3 minutes for medium or until browned and cooked to your liking. Rest for 5 minutes, then thinly slice the lamb.

In a saucepan of boiling, salted water cook carrots for 5-6 minutes until tender; in a saucepan with a bit of oil cook onions until just tender; add to carrot saucepan. Add the chickpeas and cook for 1 minute or until heated through, then drain. Toss with ginger, cumin, coriander, lemon juice, honey and remaining 2 tablespoons oil.

To serve, divide chickpea salad among plates and sprinkle with zest, then top with lamb, yogurt and extra harissa.

Organic Calf's Liver with Sage

1 calf's liver, sliced, well washed, membranes removed
1 large onion, sliced
leaves of fresh sage
butter
sea salt
pepper

In a bowl cover sliced calf's liver with boiling water. Let stand for five minutes, then drain. In a skillet cook liver and onions in butter, adding salt, pepper, and sage leaves. Do not overcook, as this destroys the critical nutrients.

Mediterranean Lamb Stew

1½ lbs. boneless lamb stew meat, (shoulder cut) or 2½ lbs. lamb shoulder chops, deboned, trimmed and cut into 1-inch chunks

2 T. extra virgin olive oil
4 tsp. ground cumin
1 T. ground coriander
2 T. minced cilantro leaves
¼ tsp. cayenne pepper
½ tsp. sea salt
1 tsp. onion powder

1 large yellow or white onion, chopped
1 28 oz. can diced tomatoes
¾ cup reduced-sodium chicken broth
3 cloves garlic, minced
1 15-oz. or 19-oz. can chickpeas, rinsed
8 oz. baby organic spinach
handful fresh green beans, stemmed, cut in one-inch pieces (optional)

Place lamb in a 4-quart or larger slow cooker. Mix oil, cumin, coriander, cayenne, sea salt, and onion powder in a small bowl. Coat the lamb with the spice paste and toss to coat well. Top with onion. In a medium saucepan over medium-high heat bring tomatoes, broth, and garlic to a simmer. Cover and cook until the lamb is very tender, 3 to 4 hours on high or 5½ to 6 hours on low, adding green beans towards the end of the cooking (about a half hour before done). Skim or blot any visible fat from the surface of the stew. Mash ½ cup chickpeas with a fork in a small bowl. Stir the mashed and whole chickpeas into the stew, along with spinach and chopped cilantro leaves. Cover and cook on high until the spinach is wilted, about 5 minutes.

Natural Beef Meat Loaf

2 pounds grass-fed or organic ground beef
2 egg yolks
4 T. parsley, minced fine
½ tsp. pepper
2 T. organic butter
1 tsp. onion juice
¼ cup oat bran tomato sauce
2 T. of chili sauce
1 package frozen peas, thawed
2 tsp. salt
parsley for garnish

Combine all of the ingredients except the tomato sauce and peas. Shape in a loaf. Butter a loaf pan, and place meat in pan. Bake in a moderate oven (350 degrees F) for 1 hour. Remove from loaf pan onto heated platter. Garnish with sprigs of parsley. Serve with tomato sauce and warmed green peas, to which a dab of butter is added when served.

Turkey Meat Loaf

1 T. extra virgin olive oil or red palm oil
1 large onion, chopped (1½ cups)
2 garlic cloves, minced
2 T. small capers
¾ tsp. sea salt, divided
½ tsp. pepper, divided
contents 3 OregaMax capsules (optional but greatly adds to the taste)
HerbSorb spice mix, ½ tsp.
⅓ cup fat-free, low-sodium chicken broth
3 tablespoons unsweetened (or honey-sweetened) ketchup, divided
1¾ pounds ground organic turkey, 97% lean
½ cup oat bran
1 large organic egg, lightly beaten
1 large organic egg white, lightly beaten

Preheat oven to 375°. Heat oil in medium skillet over medium heat. Add onion and cook, stirring frequently, until soft (5 minutes) Add garlic, ¼ tsp. salt, and ¼ tsp. pepper; cook, stirring, 1 minute. Stir in broth, and 1 T. ketchup; transfer mixture to a large bowl, and cool.

Add turkey, oat bran, capers, egg, egg white, and remaining ½ tsp. salt and ¼ tsp. pepper, along with HerbSorb and OregaMax, if available, to mixture in bowl, and mix well. (Mixture will be very moist)

Cover a baking sheet with aluminum foil, and coat lightly with cooking spray. Form the turkey mixture into a loaf, and place on the pan. Brush meat loaf evenly with remaining 2 tablespoons ketchup. Bake 1 hour or until thermometer inserted into center registers 170°. Let meat loaf stand five minutes before serving.

Curried Organic Lamb

3 T. organic butter
1 T. extra virgin olive oil
2 onions, chopped
6 celery sticks, chopped

1 clove garlic, chopped
2 cups lean diced organic lamb meat from shoulder or leg
1 /4 cup lamb broth or canned consomme
sea salt and pepper
2 T. raisins
3 T. diced mango
1 organic egg
2 T. organic heavy cream
1 T. gluten-free oat flour (or rice flour, if this isn't available)
3 tsp. curry powder dissolved in a half cup water
1 vegetable bouillon cube dissolved in same water, above

In a Dutch oven melt butter (or use a deep skillet). Add onions, garlic, and celery; cook for 5 minutes, stirring occasionally. Sprinkle olive oil over lamb. Add lamb, broth, seasonings, raisins, and mango. Cover. Allow to come to a hard boil. Then, reduce the heat and simmer 20 to 30 minutes or until meat is done. Just prior to serving beat egg and cream mixed with flour. Add curry-vegetable cube liquid; stir until thickened but do not let boil. Serve over wild or brown rice, if desired.

Italian Omelet

Filling:
4 T. organic butter
1 small red onion, finely chopped
1 medium tomato, peeled and chopped
1 T. chopped green pepper

Omelet:
3 organic eggs
2 oz. (⅓ cup) cooked pasta
salt and pepper
2 tablespoons grated Parmesan cheese
basil leaves

Prepare filling before making omelet. Melt 2 tablespoons butter in a small saucepan over low heat. Add onion and cook, stirring occasionally, 2 minutes. Stir in tomato and green pepper. Cover and cook 10 minutes.

Preheat broiler. In a small bowl, beat eggs until just mixed. Stir in pasta. Season with salt and pepper.

Set 7 inch omelet pan over low heat to become thoroughly hot. Add remaining butter to pan. When butter is sizzling but not brown, pour in egg mixture. Using a fork or spatula, draw mixture from sides to middle of pan, allowing uncooked egg to run underneath. Repeat two or three times until egg rises slightly and becomes fluffy. Cook until golden-brown underneath and top is slightly runny, about 2 minutes. Spread filling over half the omelet. Fold over and sprinkle with Parmesan. Broil just long enough to melt cheese, about 30 seconds. To serve, cut in half and garnish with basil. Serves 2.

Eggs & Salsa, Mexican style

3 organic eggs
1 T. spicy cheese, Monterrey Jack or other
3 T. salsa
2 T. green peppers finely diced
2 T. onions, finely minced
dash cayenne pepper
salt and pepper to taste
2 T. red palm oil or extra virgin olive oil

In a skillet heat the oil, then cook vegetables and onions with spices until just tender. Then, scramble eggs, adding pepper and salt and topping with salsa and cheese.

Spinach-Feta Cheese Omelet

1 T. extra virgin olive oil or red palm oil
¼ red onion thinly sliced
1 clove garlic finely chopped
fresh organic spinach, about 8 cups packed, stems removed, leaves washed
zest of 1 lemon
2 tsp. chopped fresh dill
6 free range or organic eggs beaten
¼ cup water

organic or grass-fed butter
1 ounce goat's feta cheese crumbled

In a medium-sized non-stick skillet heat ½ T. of oil; add the onion, ⅛ tsp. salt, and a pinch of pepper. Over medium heat saute for 4 to 5 minutes or until the onion is tender, then add the garlic and cook for 1 minute. Transfer to a bowl and set aside.

Heat the remaining ½ T. oil in the skillet and wilt the spinach with ¼ tsp. salt over high heat. Transfer to a colander, drain, and cool. Using your hands, squeeze out the excess moisture and coarsely chop. Add the spinach to the onions along with the lemon zest and dill. Add salt and pepper to taste. The filling should be well seasoned.

Season the eggs with ¼ tsp. salt and a few pinches of pepper; add the water and whisk. Melt the butter in a seasoned omelet pan. When the butter is hot, add half the egg mixture. With a spatula, move the eggs toward the center of the pan as they begin to stick on the edges. Tilt the pan so that the entire surface is covered again with wet eggs. As the eggs begin to set, place half the vegetable mixture in the center, then sprinkle with half the feta. Gently fold the omelet over and turn it out onto a plate. Repeat with the second omelet.

Organic Steak and Tomato Casserole

2 T. organic butter
1 pound round steak
1 small minced onion
1 small clove garlic, minced
a few drops of Oreganol P73 oil
½ tsp. or more sea salt
dash or two pepper
1 cup whole canned tomatoes
1 No. 2 can organic peas or 1 cup fresh peas
tsp. or more extra virgin olive oil

Mix olive oil with oregano oil; rub round steak well. This will help tenderize it. Chop meat into cubes. Melt butter, add onion and garlic;

saute´over low heat until tender. Add meat and keep turning with a fork until well browned, that is all the red color is gone from it. Add salt, pepper, and tomatoes; cook for 20 minutes. Drain peas if using canned peas, and put half of them in greased casserole (small to medium-sized casserole is needed). Cover with meat sauce and top with remaining peas. Dot with extra butter and any unused olive oil-oregano oil mixture. Bake at 350 degrees for 25 minutes.

Pan-Fried Browned White Fish of Any Kind in Herb Butter

4 to 5 small fish, ideally with skin on
sea salt and pepper
red sour grape powder (Resvital powder, if available)
4 T. organic butter
2 T. freshly squeezed lemon juice
2 T. finely chopped parsley
1 T. finely chopped tarragon (if available)
a bit of paprika
2 T. organic herb butter

Whip parsley and tarragon into softened butter, with a hint of paprika; set aside.

Season the fish with salt, paprika, and pepper. In a non-stick frying pan heat herbal butter and slide fish to fry to golden finish (about 5 minutes on each side). When the fish are fried and tender, switch them over to a hot platter and place lemon juice on them (use about half the reserved juice). In the frying pan put herb butter and let it come to a boil. It will begin to foam as the butter/lemon juice mixture interacts with the heat and will give a delicious taste.

Double-Decker King Oscar Sardine Sandwich

6 King Oscar sardines
2 slices gluten-free bread
2 slices all-natural cheese
4 slices tomatoes
Romaine lettuce leaf, soft green part

mustard
curry powder

On each slice of bread spread mustard but not too much to make the bread soggy; sprinkle with a hint of curry powder. Place a slice of cheese on each bread piece. Fit carefully the tomatoes slices on top, then adding the sardines, three on each bread piece, then putting the lettuce on one side. Eat as is or put in broiler-type oven, with a distance of three inches between the sandwich and the heat. Serve hot (the hot form is quite delicious and is the preferred type).

Greenwich Roll-Ups

4 organic smaller, tender collard leaves
nut butter or nut butters of your choice
finely chopped carrots and celery
grapefruit sections, membranes removed, salted
diced red sweet peppers
diced avocadoes
sprouts of your choice
humus as a dressing (optional)
sea salt
toothpicks

Cut the tough end of the collards, while also shaving off some of the cords in the center (makes it easier to roll). Spread with nut butter and then humus, then layer on sprouts, then chopped veggies, sprinkling with salt to taste. Roll up, then secure with toothpicks.

Beef Bacon Flavored Brussel Sprouts

6 slices grass fed beef bacon (or turkey bacon if available)
1 organic onion, chopped
1½ pounds organic raw brussels sprouts (not frozen), trimmed, small left whole, larger sprouts halved
1 clove of organic garlic, minced
2 T. organic full fat butter

parmesan cheese by taste
sea salt and fresh ground pepper by taste

Brown beef bacon in a medium skillet over medium high heat. Remove bacon to a paper towel lined plate. Add 2 tablespoons of butter to the bacon grease in the pan and let it melt. Add onions and garlic to the pan and sauté to 2 minutes. Add Brussels sprouts. Season with salt and pepper. Cook Brussels sprouts 2 to 3 minutes until they begin to brown or until tender. Chop up natural beef bacon and add it back to the pan for 3 to 5 minutes. Transfer sprouts to a serving dish with a slotted spoon and top with parmesan cheese.

VEGETABLES AND SIDE DISHES

Organic Carrot 'n Pea Vegetable Patties

3 T. extra virgin olive oil
4 cups grated organic carrots
1½ cups white onion, chopped
2 cloves garlic, minced
2 tsp. HerbSorb seasoning (or Herbamere seasoning)
contents of two OregaMax capsules (if available)
½ tsp. or more sea salt
2 cups frozen organic peas, thawed
1 cup rice bran
3 extra large or large eggs
½ cup organic milk or rice milk

In a large non-stick skillet heat one T. oil on medium- to medium-high heat. Add onion and cook, stirring frequently until softened. Add garlic, spices, again stirring often; cook for another two minutes. Add in carrots. Cover, reducing heat to medium or medium-low; cook for at least five minutes. Let cool slightly. Add in peas and rice bran; cook for an additional minute. In a bowl add egg and milk, whisking together. Stir in carrot mixture. Form the mixture into patties about ¾ inch thick (about 10 to 12 patties). Add the remaining oil to the skillet. On medium heat cook as many patties as will fit for about five to six minutes on each side. Serve patties with tomato-based sauce or salsa. Note: this recipe was modified from an original one by chef Carol DiPirro, whose Facebook fan page is: Chilly Peppers.

Sardined Stuffed Tomato Halves

4 small to medium organic tomatoes (use the Roma type, if available)
2 T. butter
6 to 8 sardines
1 tsp. anchovy paste
few grains cayenne
½ tsp. or more sea salt
contents of one OregaMax capsule (if available)
4 T. whipped cream

Remove skin of tomatoes, cut in half crosswise, scoop out, leaving only the shell: chill. Cream butter, add sardines, paste, salt, OregaMax, cayenne and beat lightly with a fork, carefully folding in whipped cream. sprinkle with dried parsley and paprika, if desired. Delicious and nutritious, a good source of omega 3 fatty acids.

BetaPalmed Gluten-Free Toast*

4 pieces gluten-free bread
2 T. BetaPalm or CocaPalm
contents one or two OregaMax capsules

In a large skillet heat gluten-free bread in oil over medium-high heat. Cook until desired crispness on each side.

Mashed Potato Puffs

2 cups cold mashed potatoes
¼ tsp. pepper
2 T. organic butter, melted
2 organic eggs, separated

¼ tsp. salt
6 T. cream
oat bran
butter

Mix the cold mashed potatoes, melted butter, some salt and pepper to a fine, light, and creamy texture: then, add eggs, well beaten, separately, and the cream. Beat it all well and lightly together. Shape the mixture into suitably sized portions and roll in oat bran. Place in a greased pan with butter over each puff, and brown in the oven (400 to 450 degrees F), turning once.

Roasted Whole Head Cauliflower

1 T. extra virgin olive oil
1 head organic cauliflower
1½ cups plain organic Greek whole fat yogurt
1 lime, zested and juiced
1 T. chili powder
1 T. paprika
1 T. cumin
1 T. garlic powder
1 tsp. curry powder
2 tsp. sea salt
contents 4 OregaMax capsules (if available)

Preheat oven to 400° and lightly grease a small baking sheet with oil. Trim the base of cauliflower to remove green leaves and woody stem. Clean the florette carefully.

In a medium bowl combine the yogurt with the lime zest and juice, chile powder, paprika, cumin, garlic powder, curry powder, salt, and pepper. Dunk the cauliflower into the bowl and use a brush or your hands to smear the marinade evenly over its surface (excess marinade can be stored in the refrigerator in an airtight container for up to 3 days and used with meat, fish, or other veggies. Place cauliflower on the prepared baking sheet and roast until the surface is dry and lightly browned, 30 to 40 minutes. The marinade will make a crust on the surface of the cauliflower. Let cool for 10 minutes before cutting into wedges. serve as is or, preferably, with romaine lettuce salad.

Herb-Buttered Parsnip Strips

3 T. melted butter
1 T. finely minced parsley
1 T. very finely minced onion
paprika as desired
contents 2 OregaMax capsules, if available (greatly adds to the taste)
2 medium-sized parsnips
½ tsp. sea salt
¼ tsp. black pepper

Put parsley and finely minced onion in butter. Pare the parsnips and then slice in the large-sized long slicer hole. Make into long strips, thin as wallpaper. In a small casserole grease it and pile parsnips into it gently, dot with butter mixture generously and then season with salt, pepper, and paprika. Bake for 30 minutes in a moderate 350-degree oven

SOUPS AND SALADS

Pureéd Fish Creamy Soup

1 small onion, minced
1 quart organic whole fat milk
2 T. heavy cream (optional)
4 T. unsalted butter
4 T. brown rice or gluten-free oat flour
½ tsp. paprika
⅛ tsp. pepper
1 T. finely minced fresh parsley
2 cups cooked fish

In a pot scald minced onion in small amount of milk. Melt in butter, and blend in flour, salt, and pepper. Add milk with cream mixed in gradually, stirring constantly. Force fish through a sieve, and add to sauce. Serve hot garnished with paprika and parsley.

Organic Liver and Dandelion Salad

4 handfuls wild or commercial dandelion leaves
½ pound organic calf's or beef liver
4 T. extra virgin olive oil
2 medium onions, minced
2 T. balsamic vinegar (use apple cider vinegar, if this isn't available)
2 T. fresh parsley, minced
sea salt
pepper

Chill a serving plate. Clean dandelion leaves thoroughly, and arrange on serving plate. Cut liver into slices. In a skillet on medium heat cook onions for about two minutes. Add livers and cook until firm but still pink inside. Season with sea salt and pepper. Place liver slices on dandelion leaves, topping with bits of parsley. Pour remaining oil, along with vinegar, over livers and serve.

Fresh Wild Rice Organic Chicken Soup

This recipe is a modification of Chef Emeril Lagasse's delicious chicken soup recipe with brown rice. The spice base, here, is somewhat different. Plus, turnips are added as a vegetable, and the option is given to use red palm oil as a sautéing agent instead of olive oil.

2 T. extra virgin olive oil or red palm oil
1 whole chicken, about 3 pounds, boned with skin on (save bones and carcass)
1 cup purple or yellow carrots, diced
½ cup turnips, chopped in cubes
2 cups onions, chopped
½ cup celery, chopped
¼ cup green onions, diced
2 T. minced garlic
¼ cup fresh parsley leaves, minced

1 cup fresh spinach leaves, chopped
4 bay leaves
contents 4 OregaMax capsules (if available) or T. dried oregano
1 T. garlic powder
1 T. onion powder
½ T. black pepper
1 T. paprika
2½ T. sea salt
⅓ pound wild rice
3 quarts chicken stock

Mix all spices together and get ready for use. In a large pot heat extra virgin olive oil. Season chicken with all spices and add to oil; add bones and carcass. Sauté for about five minutes; remove carcass and bones. Add onions, celery green onions, garlic, carrots, parsley, along with bay leaves. Season with more spice mixture. Sauté vegetables for about 4 minutes, adding chopped vegetables and spinach; cook for about a minute. Now, add the stock and wild rice, and bring to a boil. Simmer uncovered for about 20 to 25 minutes or until rice is thoroughly tender.

Wild Dandelion Mediterranean Salad

Find an area with wild spring dandelions which is not sprayed or tainted. Pick an ice cream bucket full. Clean and refrigerate, reserving 4 cups for the recipe:

4 cups wild dandelion leaves
1 large cucumber, peeled and cut into wedges
8 to 12 organic cherry tomatoes

Dressing:
2 T. minced red onions
1 T. minced parsley
2 OregaMax capsules, emptied
1 T. fresh lemon juice
4 T. extra virgin olive oil
2 T. balsamic vinegar

1 T. pomegranate molasses (PomaMax)
pinch or two of sea salt

Toss wild dandelions with cucumbers and tomatoes. Mix salad dressing ingredients. In bowls placed tossed salad, and drizzle with dressing.

Rich Romaine and Feta Cheese Salad

14 spears of Romaine lettuce, chopped
¼ cup crumbled sheep goat cheese
2 T. minced red onion
2 T. minced red sweet pepper
4 radishes, sliced
2 or 3 T. extra virgin olive oil
2 T. balsamic vinegar
2 tsp. pomegranate syrup (PomaMax)
½ tsp. capers
sea salt to taste

In a good sized bowl add lettuce with radishes, onion, peppers, and capers. Then add feta cheese topped with extra virgin olive oil, balsamic vinegar, and pomegranate syrup. Add sea salt to taste.

Super-Rich Beefy Borsch Soup

1 cup tomatoes, fresh or canned
2 cups shredded beets
4 cups water
1 medium onion, cut in small pieces
½ lb. lean organic range-fed beef, cut in chunky cubes
1 tsp. fresh lemon juice
1 tsp. raw honey
½ tsp. sea salt
4 whole organic eggs
sour cream

Through a fine sieve, strain tomatoes over beets. Add water, onion and meat and simmer for 30 minutes. Add lemon juice, honey and salt. Boil

30 minutes longer. Beat eggs and add them to the borsch a little at a time, stirring well with each addition. Serve while very hot, topped with sour cream.

Extra-Rich Squash Soup

4 cups organic milk
1 T. minced onion
¼ bay leaf
½ tsp. Herbsorb spice mix
2 cups cooked, strained squash
3 T. organic butter
3 T. gluten-free oat flour or brown rice flour
2 vegetarian bouillon cubes
1½ tsp. sea salt
dash of cayenne pepper
2 T. fresh chopped parsley or 1 T. dried parsley

Scald milk with onion and bay leaf, strain and add squash. Melt butter and blend in flour, salt, HerbSorb, bouillon cubes, and cayenne. Add milk mixture gradually, while stirring constantly. Cook for 5 minutes, and serve garnished with parsley.

White Radish Soup

Like carrots, radishes have antiseptic properties. Thus, they make an ideal addition to salad. Much of their antiseptic powers is retained even after cooking. Here is a rare recipe for radish soup:

1 lb. white radishes scraped and cut, tops removed (reserve the best pieces of the tops, if unwilted; clean thoroughly to remove all sand and grit)
5 cups organic turkey or chicken stock
1 tsp. curry powder
1 cup organic half and half
1 tsp. horseradish
some dry mustard
a bit of dried or fresh parsley
tsp. or two chopped chives

In a saucepan combine radishes with enough chicken stock to cover (2 to 3 cups). Bring to a boil. Cook until tender over moderate heat, about 10 to 20 minutes. Puree; add 2 more cups stock and curry plus mustard and horseradish. Stir in half and half. Soup may be served hot or chilled. Shortly before serving add parsley and chives.

Organic Minty Cantaloupe Soup

2½ cups freshly squeezed juice from organic oranges or tangerines
½ tsp. cinnamon
2 T. lime juice
1 large ripe organic cantaloupe, skinned and seeded
Mint sprigs, stems removed

Be sure to chop cantaloupe coarsely in chunks. In a blender or food processor combine all ingredients and blend into a puree. Chill and serve garnished with mint and, if desired, sprinkled with cinnamon and nutmeg.

Garden Soup

8 cups chopped organic Romaine or other lettuce
½ cup chopped organic green pepper
6 green onions, finely chopped
1 medium cucumber, peeled and chopped
1 cup chopped parsley
1 large clove garlic, minced
1 qt. organic buttermilk
⅓ cup each organic sour cream and heavy cream
2 T. fresh lemon juice
2 tsp. sea salt
contents two OregaMax capsules (if available)
a few drops Tabasco sauce

In a bowl combine greens, garlic, green onions, and buttermilk; puree in batches. In a separate bowl mix together cream, sour cream, and lemon juice; stir into garden soup. Add salt and Tabasco sauce to taste.

Special Chopped Sardine Salad

3 cans sardines, ideally King Oscar in olive oil
6 radishes, chopped (chop a few greens and add in if firm and unwilted; wash well)
1 medium carrot, chopped
1 medium onion, chopped
12 cherry tomatoes, halved
2 T. extra virgin olive oil
2 or 3 T. balsamic vinegar
1 T. Mediterranean pomegranate syrup (PomaMax)
sea salt to taste

Add together all vegetables. Cut up sardines and top with extra virgin olive oil, vinegar and pomegranate syrup. Season to taste.

Traditional Greek Salad

½ cup crumbled goat's or sheep's feta
½ cup green or black olives, pitted, halved
1 medium-to-large red onion, sliced
½ head iceberg lettuce
½ bunch Romaine lettuce
2 cups cherry tomatoes, sliced in half
1 can anchovy fillets

Dressing:
1 cup extra virgin olive oil
¼ cup vinegar
2 T. freshly squeezed lemon juice
1 T. wild oregano (or contents of 5 OregaMax capsules)
sea salt and pepper to taste

In a large bowl combine all ingredients (except dressing); shake back-and-forth well. In a separate container mix dressing. Pour over salad and serve.

Organic Chicken Nut Soup

1 cup celery, chopped
4 cups organic chicken stock
½ tsp. Herbsorb spice mix
sea salt and pepper
1 organic egg, beaten
1 T. rice flour or gluten-free oat flour
1 cup whole organic milk
⅓ cup ground nut meats of your choice
whipped cream
2 T. minced fresh parsley
Pumpkinol whole food Austrian pumpkinseed Oil

Add stock and celery in a pot and cook celery until tender. Combine, egg, flour, Herbsorb, nut meats, and milk—beat well. Add to stock gradually and cook for 5 minutes, stirring constantly. Season with salt and pepper and top with Pumpkinol, if available, along with whipped cream and parsley.

Beet & Onion Salad

I lb. beets cooked, peeled, cut into thin julienne strips
2 shallots, finely chopped
¼ cup extra virgin olive oil
lettuce leaves of your choice
½ small onion, thinly sliced, separated into rings
1 T. chopped parsley

In a glass dish, mix beets, shallots and extra virgin olive oil. Let marinate 2 hours. Line a serving dish with lettuce leaves; spoon in salad and scatter onions on top. Garnish with parsley and serve. Makes 4 to 6 servings.

Fruit Salad with Coconut Lime Dressing

Granny Smith apple slices
Bosc pear slices
grapes

dressing:

2 ozs. creamed coconut
2 T. boiling water
1 tsp. grated ginger root
2 tsp. finely grated lime peel
1 T. fresh lime juice
1 tsp. raw honey
¼ cup full fat yogurt

In a small bowl, cover coconut with boiling water. Stir until smooth. Cover and refrigerate until cold. Stir in ginger root, lime peel and juice, raw honey and yogurt until well blended. Cover with plastic wrap and refrigerate until needed. Makes ⅔ cup. Serve over fruit.

Parsley Root and Parsnip Salad

6 medium parsley roots, ends cut off, cut into one-inch chunks, halved
2 medium parsnips, ends cut off, cut into bite-sized chunks
8 cherry tomatoes, halved
one half medium red onion, diced
2 T. chopped parsley
2 T. extra virgin olive oil
2 T. balsamic vinegar
pine nuts (optional)
sea salt

In a bowl add all vegetables, then extra virgin olive oil, vinegar, pine nuts, and sea salt. Toss and serve.

Popeye Salad

Like Popeye seemed to know, downing cans of spinach can make a person more powerful. This sweet leafy green is literally packed with nutrients, including vitamins A, C, and E, folic acid and calcium plus a goodly amount of potassium. It also has a rich supply of iron. Extremely versatile, spinach can be eaten fresh, steamed, boiled, sauteed or baked into a wide range of dishes. Use it as often as possible on this nutrient-rich program, whether raw or cooked.

8 cups fresh, organic baby spinach
1 hard boiled egg, preferably organic, sliced in half lengthwise
6 olives
½ cup goat's or sheep's feta cheese, crumbled
1 cup whole cherry tomatoes, chopped
1 cup garbanzo beans
a few slices of avocado
2 T. red bell pepper, sliced
3 T. extra virgin olive oil
2 T. fresh lemon juice
sea salt to taste

Divide spinach onto two plates and top each serving with half the remaining ingredients.

Special Red and Green Cabbage Salad

1 cup shredded red cabbage (note: if red cabbage is unavailable, double the amount of green cabbage)
1 cup shredded green cabbage
½ cup grated carrot
⅓ green pepper, sliced
1 tart or sour apple, sliced
2 T. chopped red or yellow onion
½ cup chopped celery
¼ cup chopped dill pickle
extra virgin olive oil and balsamic vinegar
sea salt
paprika

Mix all ingredients together with as much vinegar and olive oil as desired and season with salt and paprika. Place on lettuce leaves and serve.

Tomato-Cucumber Salad

Tomatoes and cucumbers are cooling. Celery boosts the adrenal glands. This is an ideal salad for summer or hot months yet is also good, all year long.

2 tomatoes, cut in eighths
½ cucumber, diced
3 red or white radishes, diced
red onion, diced (a T. or two)
1 celery stick, diced
a few English walnut meats
apple cider vinegar and oil of your choice (walnut oil would be ideal)

Mix together all ingredients and toss. Serve chilled.

DRINKS AND SMOOTHIES

Pomegranate Bubbly Surprise

6 T. Mediterranean sour pomegranate syrup
1 quart sparkling mineral water
ice, if desired

Mix and serve chilled. Ideal for supporting the health of the heart.

Raw Egg Super Shake

2 organic raw eggs
1 T. Purely-B
handful frozen berries
1 tsp. wild baobab powder
½ cup full fat yogurt
water or berry juice to desired thickness

Blend until creamy and consume as a breakfast or between meals power shake.

Raw Egg Almond Milk Carob Shake

2 organic raw eggs, whether whole or the yolks only
1 T. or more Purely-B
handful organic frozen berries

1 tsp. wild baobab powder
almond milk to desired thickness

Blend until creamy and consume as a breakfast or between meals power shake

Organic Carrot 'n Dandelion Flush/Cleanse Juice

12 raw organic carrots, cleaned and ends cut off
bunch organic dandelion leaves (or wild spring dandelion leaves)

In a juicer juice vegetables. Drink as a cleanse, half in the morning and the other half at night. Both carrots and dandelion leaves possess diuretic properties. Dandelion has strong cleansing capacities for the bowel, blood, and liver, while carrot specializes in cleansing the kidneys and intestinal tract.

DESSERTS

Greek Yogurt Fruit Parfait

2 cups whole milk organic Greek yogurt
ground flaxseed
half banana, sliced
a few organic strawberries, sliced
T. raw honey

In a sundae glass add yogurt and make a surround with bananas and strawberries. Sprinkle with ground flaxseed and top with honey.

Fat-Rich Blueberry Dream

1 cup organic fresh blueberries
1 small carton organic full-fat cottage cheese
1 pint organic full-fat sour cream
2 T. raw honey (wild oregano or another)

Mix blueberries with raw honey; this recipe is not excessively sweet and relies on the fat for taste and richness. Combine cottage cheese with the sour cream, folding the cheese into the cream until nicely blended. Pile the berries in the middle, and serve in a nice bowl, the berries showing through the creamy whiteness.

Creamed Fruit ala Cottage Cheese

1 cup creamed organic full fat cottage cheese
4 T. dates, minced (use wet scissors to cut into bits)
½ sliced banana
½ cup crushed pineapple
1 cup organic heavy cream, whipped
2 T. liquid honey or all-natural, real maple syrup
salt (a few grains)

In a large bowl combine cottage cheese and dates plus banana and crushed pineapple, then the sweetener and salt. Then, whipped cream; fold cream into the mixture. Pour into freezing tray and freeze for about 5 hours or until fruit mixture is nice and firm.

Blackberry Super Frozen Yogurt

⅔ cup frozen organic blueberries
3 cups fresh or frozen and partially thawed organic or wild blackberries
½ cup water
3 T. raw honey
2 T. lemon juice
1 T. organic or grass-fed butter
2 cups plain 2% reduced-fat organic Greek yogurt

Combine the first 5 ingredients in a small saucepan. Bring mixture to a boil. Reduce heat to medium-low; gently boil 10 minutes or until sauce thickens. Stir in butter. Spoon ½ cup yogurt into each of 4 bowls; top each serving with about ¼ cup sauce.

Diced Fruit 'n Nut Yogurt Iced Surprise

2 cups full fat yogurt
½ cup frozen organic blueberries
1 cup frozen organic strawberries
½ cup frozen blackberries
walnuts, pine nuts, and filberts to mix in (if pine nuts are unavailable, use chunks of pecans)
raw honey to taste

In a bowl add yogurt, then berries, then nuts and honey; mix as well as possible. Eat as an icy treat or let thaw out and consume an hour or so later.

Pineapple and Melon Cocktail

ripe melon of your choice
diced fresh or canned pineapple
freshly squeezed lemon juice
a few mint leaves
a hint of fresh ginger
raw honey to taste

Mix fruit together in a bowl, being sure to cut both into small easy-to-serve pieces. Add in a tablespoon or so of fresh lemon juice, along with honey and mint leaves plus ginger, well sliced or chopped (you can dust with ginger powder if fresh isn't available). Chill until cold and serve, piled into clear fruit compote cups.

Chapter Sixteen

The Lyme Child

The "Lyme child" should never exist. How can a child's entire life, or a teenager's life, be corrupted by a biting insect? How dreadful it is for children to contract what is nothing other than a form of weaponized syphilis. Yet, it is true; it happens by the tens of thousands every year, and this is in the United States alone.

Moorcraft has brought out good points on the difference in the presentation of Lyme in children versus adults. In the former the most common features are surely novel, which include sleep disorders as possibly the main symptom, including nightmares and new onset bedwetting. There may be, he notes, an increase in daytime urinary urgency as well as frequency. One bizarre symptom, which, by the way, may also happen to adults, is " discomfort when being touched." Additionally, "Children often complain of headaches, mild to debilitating." There are surely, he has made clear, also digestive disorders, stomach ache, intestinal spasms, and more. There may be rather abrupt alterations in personality, which might include obvious changes in behavior and even temper tantrums and outbursts. Says Moorcraft, incredibly, "once happy children become irritable and sad." Even though this may be due to just the Lyme spirochete, it could be a sign of multiple infections. In fact, he writes, if they develop an additional constellation of symptoms, for instance, abrupt changes in mood "to the point that they are depressed, anxious, psychotic and even suicidal, then, co-infection by bartonella must be considered." Furthermore, previously "normal, even gregarious, children as a result of the infestation may become sheepish and withdrawn." They may "develop odd, repetitive behaviors and/or tics. When several of these symptoms are seen in the same child, they may be misdiagnosed with autism." It is, therefore, a challenge to make a definitive diagnosis of Lyme, in particular when it mimics the standard symptoms of attention deficit and ADHD. Investigators often consider the plausibility of vaccine damage and may miss the fact that it is Lyme that is the primary source of their physiological collapse. The vaccines do, though, play a preeminent role by weakening the system, making the child more vulnerable to the Lyme spirochete onslaught.

Moorcroft is in the epicenter of this catastrophe, the State of Connecticut itself. There, he has found, the disease is truly epidemic and severe, perhaps more severe than elsewhere in the country.

Yet, will the child cases be more readily realized? A thorough history might resolve this. If there is a history of onset somehow related to outdoor activity and/or if the condition originated after, for instance, age three, where such activity might be expected, this may be a revelation. Dogs in the family that would be in close contact with potentially infected children could also be an indication. Too, if the parents had suffered from known Lyme disease, surely there is a possibility of intrauterine transfer.

Even so, children are truly highly vulnerable. The tiny tick nymph readily attacks them and is only rarely seen for preventive purposes. Unless they are carefully inspected, then, that nymph will go on to infect them. The existence of a bullseye rash or some other sudden onset rash would help, yet it only occurs in at most one of three cases. Single joint swelling or inflammation is a key sign, if it is recognized as such.

Lyme in children is a major issue from a statistical point of view. Nearly one fourth of all US cases are in children. This means that, yearly, 75,000 new childhood cases develop. Many of these cases are clearly misdiagnosed as other conditions, for instance, ADD, ADHD, Crohn's disease, multiple sclerosis, Bell's palsy, chronic fatigue syndrome, fibromyalgia, juvenile arthritis, and others.

Says C. Ray Jones, M.D., who specializes in Lyme treatment in children, "Of the more than 5000 children I've treated 240 have been *born with the disease*." He also determined that some of the child cases *contracted it through breast feeding*.

Jones has more than this to say about childhood Lyme. While, he notes, most physicians believe that the disease presents nearly always with a standard set of physical symptoms, such as fever, rash, and joint pain, Jones has observed that in children it can have a far wider presentation, which may include mental symptoms.

Originally treating the disease's symptoms in the late 1960s, before it was officially recognized by most medical professionals, it was Jones who offered his own clinical cases to researchers who made the disease publically known. This included Yale professor Allen Steere, who has been at the center of a controversy versus patients with chronic Lyme disease. For instance, Jones is certain the chronic form of the disease is pandemic, while Steere disputes this. It was Steere, among others, who propounded that the disease is readily cured with three to six weeks of antibiotics, even though there is much evidence to the contrary. Hostility from Steere and others has led to what appears to be a plot against Dr. Jones. He is being attacked and 'disciplined,' as well as fined, by the Connecticut medical board. Yet, says Jones in an interview with YaleDailyNews.com, "I'm not being disciplined, I'm being harassed."

One of his other adversaries, Eugene Shapiro, a pediatrician at the Yale School of Medicine, has gone so far as to attack anything associated with chronic Lyme, including its very existence: "As for chronic Lyme, there is no definition and I believe there is *no such entity*," said Shapiro.

Yet, Jones' work speaks for itself. When this article was posted online, "Amid Controversy, Children Saved," people gave revelation of their dire circumstances before undergoing the doctor's care, including one with the moniker, LymeFamily:

> Dr. Jones is a walking, breathing saint. My daughter would not be at gymnastics, school, or playing the piano if it weren't for him. I can only imagine she would be in a wheelchair and possibly admitted to a psychiatric hospital without his care. Our pediatrician denied treatment for her at 3 YEARS OF AGE after becoming violently ill from a tick bite. I watched her become sicker and sicker as I desperately reached out to our doctor to please help her. She would have tantrums that lasted for two hours, she was losing hair and wasting away. She lost bladder control. She couldn't walk down the stairs anymore. The list goes on. Still he would not treat her because she didn't have a bull's eye rash.

Obviously, this child was under severe attack by the Lyme bacillus, which was attacking all her body systems. This included the nervous system, that is the brain and spinal cord, as manifested by the loss of bladder control.

There is no question that in the arena of chronic Lyme disease Jones is a pioneer. Moreover, one pertinent issue is the fact that he had determined its existence long before any other, notably in the 1960s. This is, perhaps, a decade before pockets of the disease in this same state were realized. Yet, this does not preclude the biogerm origin of the condition. Tick vector research originated in Plum Island as early as the 1950s. Moreover, with the West Nile disease outbreak connected to the lab the Lyme connection to the lab still remains a strong possibility.

Antibiotics may well be required in the treatment of Lyme disease in children, whether acute or chronic. Yet, the therapy should also include the intake of the oil of wild oregano, including a super-strength form, multiple spice oil liquid complexes, the whole crude herb plus *Rhus coriaria,* the wild turmeric drops, the wild chaga drops, a high-grade probiotic supplement (Ecologic 500), fatty high vitamin A wild salmon oil, a deep-eezing rubbing oil, bone activating rubbing oil, and the juice of wild oregano. One benefit, here, is that these supplements are all liquids and/or powders. This is the minimal protocol for the assistance in eradicating the pathogens and, therefore, regaining optimal health.

Chapter Seventeen

Conclusion

No doubt, Lyme disease is an exceptionally difficult condition to cure, because of its nature: because of the nature of the arch-antagonistic germ itself. Rather than an infection readily recognized by the immune system, it is caused by a man-made germ, a mutant. It would be reasonable enough if it was a naturally occurring consequence. Surely, there would be a way for the body to deal with it. For human survival there would certainly be a natural, native mechanism to recognize it and destroy it. If not this, then, surely, there would be some simple formula, whether medical or natural-source, to deal with it. Yet, this is not to be. That's because it's not even a freak of nature but is, rather, one of human meddling, a laboratory aberration, a complete anomaly, a corruption to the extreme.

Even so, through the use of powerful natural cures in most cases the disease can be completely cured. In some cases despite the most yeoman efforts there may be residual damage. Yet, given sufficient time and effort this damage may prove reversible. This is speaking from experience. Lyme disease has proven to be the most stubborn of virtually all diseases. It takes great patience and persistence to cure it. Yet, as proven by experience it can be reversed even in the most severe and seemingly hopeless cases.

Some people are more fortunate than others. They realize that they have a tick bite and seek medical aid immediately. If the infection can be caught and halted before it gains a foothold, then, the results are usually positive. It is simply far easier to treat when it first invades, that is before it fully and thoroughly infests the body.

Even so, regardless of the medical history and scope of the disease, no one should ever give up hope on Lyme. It's merely a bacterial infection—although it may represent infections by multiple species of such bacteria, including bartonella and the bacteria-like *Mycoplasma fermentans*. Moreover, bacteria can be readily killed. Once such pathogens are killed and/or purged from the body, then good health will return. Lyme, bartonella, and mycoplasma are more difficult to kill than the typical bacteria, because they hide themselves intracellularly. Even so, given time they can be destroyed; the spice oils will eventually burn them out of the body. Moreover, they will do so just as efficiently if not more so than orthodox drugs.

No doubt, the vast majority of cases of Lyme and co-infection diseases are the result of tick bites. Yet, as has been made clear throughout this book there are other less well recognized means by which to acquire the disease. One of these is mosquito bites. Another is the bites of biting flies and also fleas as well as possibly mites. Blood transfusions can readily infect individuals with the Lyme spirochete as well as a wide range of other tick-originating germs including the protozoan babesia.

Too, as mentioned previously it has been confirmed that an infected mother can transmit the disease to her newborn child through placental transfer. Along with the Lyme spirochete, babesia, mycoplasma, and bartonella have also been transferred this way. Additionally, let it not be forgotten that the disease is transferable through sexual intercourse.

In non-endemic regions, like southeastern Texas, the cases of Lyme are on the rise. Through work by a number of M.D.s in Houston, Texas, including W.T. Harvey and his group, it was determined that the disease is being transmitted by other vectors besides ticks. For the Texas cases these vectors include fleas, mites, and mosquitoes.

Therefore, the risks for contracting Lyme are far more significant than most people realize. Says one Internet poster on a Lyme forum:

> The government knows…the blood bank is contaminated and it is sexually transmitted. I got it from my husband. We have three of the same tick-borne infections, Lyme, babesia, and mycoplasma…(We have) both been sick long term. I am unable to work for over three years…I can't wait until all people know the danger of this horrific disease, how many lives were lost to it, how many suicides were carried out because the disease tortures you 24/7. Many, many people have taken their own lives, because the pain and suffering is hideous…Chronic Lyme makes you wish for death, and you don't get it until you get it.

That 'torture' component—the agony, the hideousness, and more—is a non-issue for those who use the vigorous natural cure protocols in this book. It is merely a matter of time until the health is regenerated and those horrific symptoms are eliminated, although each case is different.

The torture, though, is universal. While the circumstances in the United States have been emphasized here, the disease may be contracted virtually anywhere in the world. Tens of thousands of cases occur yearly in Europe. Furthermore, the claim that the condition is not found in the far north Canada or in the deep South is entirely false. Though more common in the mid-to-upper Northern Hemisphere Lyme has been contracted from virtually every region of the world. Consider the work done by canlyme.com:

Lyme disease is present in most of Canada. Although Lyme infection is more common in rural areas, residents that live in urban areas are also at risk for infection. It is the migratory birds, robins and song sparrows etc. that bring this disease in each season.

No one is entirely immune. Therefore, the necessary precautions must be taken. One such precaution is to greatly bolster the powers of the immune system. Yet another is to carefully take care of the body, staying in optimal health, following a healthy and toxin-free diet. Still another is to stay active and get plenty of exercise and sunshine. The greatest precaution, though, is to take the spice oil-based supplements on a regular basis: to create a kind of antiseptic power of the blood.

Of course, another key prevention is avoid getting bit. Yet, in some cases that may prove impossible. Even so, extraordinary efforts should be taken to minimize exposure, including the wearing of the proper protective clothing and also the use of appropriate repellents. In this regard the aggressive use of Herbal Tick-X (or Herbal Bug-X for mosquitoes) will prove effective. Too, never go out in the wilderness without doing the standard technique, which is pulling the socks over the pant-legs. Women in the wilderness should always wear pants: no exceptions.

If Lyme does occur, the treatment must be aggressive and continuous, not for a few days or weeks but, rather, for several months. The infective levels of the bacteria and other germs may be killed, but they may not be completely destroyed, altering themselves into dormant forms. For Lyme this represents the cystic entity. This cyst is able to remain dormant, but when placed into an environment favorable to its growth, it often reverts to the infective form. The typical antibiotics used for Lyme, such as the penicillins, tetrayclines, and cephalosporins, are impotent against this cyst.

This is not the case with the wild spice oils. They dissolve all forms of the spirochete, whether the live, active cork-screw entity, the cyst form, or the slime-coated L-form.

Therefore, for the achievement of an absolute and long-term cure there is no other option other than the use of high-potency spice oils and other spice-based medicines. The natural remedies are the only categorical answer for Lyme. As there is no toxicity for any of the natural spice oil and/or whole food remedies mentioned in this book, they can be taken with impunity. A person can, thus, be as aggressive as is necessary in order to obliterate the Lyme spirochetes and the co-infection agents, once and for all from the body.

This has to be done. Otherwise, the germ will eventually destroy the body, causing great disease and premature death. Moreover, clearly, it is not good enough to merely take antibiotics. Surely, such drugs will not no matter how high the dose or how prolonged the treatment eradicate the Lyme bacillus in the majority of cases. Even with those taking antibiotics there must be other therapies applied, and these surely must be from the natural pharmacy.

For those who desire a therapy other than the orthodox, surely the spice oils are the most reliable modality. They are decided germicides, and thus they kill the Lyme spirochete, along with all co-infective germs. When the germ is killed or as it is being killed, then, there will be a consequence. This consequence is the relief of many if not all of the agonizing, resistant, and frightening symptoms.

In fact, it is a frightening condition. For all anyone would know the disease would eventually overcome the individual, gradually diminishing such a one, systematically corrupting the person's health. Ultimately, it would then cause a degree of corruption that is irreversible: chronic degenerative disease and premature death. Yet, this is true only in those who undergo no treatment or who exclusively rely on drug therapy as the cure.

In conquering Lyme the government will not help and is not helping. People have to take action on their own. In fact, clearly, for purposes of deception government policy has led to a worsening of the crisis. As with the West Nile outbreak the source origin of Lyme as a biogerm was made top secret: no leaks allowed.

Can it be a coincidence that both these diseases had as their epicenter areas within a small mile radius, a mere 10 miles or less, of the infamous Plum Island biogerm lab? It's all lies; no one will speak the truth about this criminal enterprise. Regardless, it cannot be a coincidence, particularly considering the fact that, for instance, West Nile is a tropical disease, and there is no way it would have naturally broken out in the New York City and Long Island areas unless it was a man-made intervention.

Hiding the truth is corrupt beyond comprehension, and all it leads to is an even greater horror and corruption. Here, the truth, the information, regarding natural cures, that is natural-source options for the treatment of Lyme, is fully revealed. It is a revelation that will never come from orthodox sources, which actually fight the public introduction of such information, even though by no means will this do any harm.

The natural remedies mentioned in this book provide powerful alternatives for Lyme victims. These are also alternatives that will prove lifesaving. If taken aggressively and consistently they will even do the untenable: eradicate the disease entirely. That is the power offered by wild nature, one that no synthetic drugs can match.

Moreover, the victims should never give up to any degree. It is crucial to stay the course. The natural medicines must be used as aggressively as necessary. Do not be shy to take large doses—as large as is needed—to eliminate this scourge from the body. As a result, ultimately, this condition will be cured.

Lyme can be defeated. Key supplements include the oil of wild oregano, juice of wild oregano, the whole crude herb complex with *Rhus coriaria*, the bone activating rubbing oil, bone activating capsules, the multiple spice dessicated oil capsules, inflammation-easing enzyme complex, and probiotics, along with, if available, teasel root extract.

No doubt, one of the most powerful, novel therapeutic approaches against this disease is to strengthen the skeletal system. The Lyme bacillis vigorously attacks this system. This is why the use of the bone-activating rubbing oil and capsules is so crucial. In the relapse involving the knee it was these supplements, along with the raw, whole food freshwater cod liver oil, that were crucial in achieving a cure. Use these as indicated, along with the dozens of other supplements mentioned and the anti-Lyme supplement system, for a complete recovery.

Also, it is essential to protect yourself in the wilderness. Follow the preventive protocols, and be sure to vigorously use the high-potency Herbal Tick-X spray.

Through the powers of wild nature Lyme can be defeated. It is the only true hope for all who have suffered so greatly from this treachery, the best path to take to achieve the ultimate cure.

Appendix A

Signs and Symptoms of Lyme Disease

- swelling in a single joint
- stiffness in a single joint
- swelling or stiffness of the knee, ankle, elbow, or shoulder
- joints which are painful to deep pressure
- achiness of the shoulders, especially upon awakening
- shoulders are weak; difficulty putting arm through shirt when dressing
- wake up with shoulder weakness or pain
- shoulders or arms ache at night
- painful elbows
- juvenile arthritis
- flu-like illness
- fever
- bullseye rash (known as erythema migrans)
- malar flush
- red ear lobes
- TMJ/jaw pain
- clicking of the TMJ
- neck pain
- back pain
- bone pain
- chills
- sweats
- tiredness
- sore throat
- hair loss
- sudden weight loss
- difficulty swallowing
- swelling around the eyes
- insomnia
- anxiety

- Tourette's syndrome
- arrhythmia
- paralysis of the face on one side (Bell's palsy)
- sensation as if existing in another world or sensation as if the brain is missing
- not feeling like the same person (an almost out of body feeling)
- surreal sensations
- emotions are out of control
- loss of focus
- sensation as if head is exploding
- feeling as if burning up
- feeling like the skin is on fire
- stiffness of the upper back
- feeling like the spine is exploding
- swelling of the lymph glands, especially in the armpit, neck, and inguinal area
- waking up with a headache
- pressure inside the head
- panicky feeling
- depression
- moodiness
- a sense of hopelessness
- neck stiffness
- sound sensitivity
- memory disorders
- brain fog
- vaginitis
- prostatitis
- sensation of being drained of all energy and power
- numbness in the feet or hands
- numbness of the arms
- paralysis of one side of the body
- full-body paralysis (rare)
- sudden outbreak of a rash
- chest pain or rib soreness
- shortness of breath
- heart palpitations

- pulse skips
- heart block
- heart murmur or valve prolapse
- nausea or vomiting
- constipation
- diarrhea
- gastritis
- abdominal cramping
- irritable bladder or bladder dysfunction
- cystitis
- muscle pain in feet
- swelling in toes
- swelling in balls of feet
- ankle pain
- burning in feet
- shin splints
- stiffness of the joints
- migrating muscle pain
- migrating joint pain
- muscle cramps
- twitching of the face, eyelids or other muscles
- headache
- tingling
- numbness
- burning or stabbing sensations
- dizziness
- poor balance
- increased motion sickness
- light-headedness
- wooziness
- difficulty walking
- tremor
- confusion, difficulty in thinking or with concentration or reading
- forgetfulness
- poor short term memory

- disorientation (getting lost, going to wrong place)
- difficulty with speech
- double or blurry vision
- eye pain
- ear pain
- blindness
- increased floaters
- increased sensitivity to buzzing or ringing in ears
- deafness
- seizures
- low blood pressure.
- mood swings
- violent outburst
- irritability
- wake up too early in the morning
- disturbed sleeping patterns
- personality changes
- obsessive compulsive disorder (OCD)
- paranoia
- hallucinations
- testicular pain or pelvic pain
- menstrual irregularity
- sexual dysfunction
- loss of libido

Signs and Symptoms of Bartonella

- neurological symptoms out of proportion to other symptoms of Lyme
- fever
- fatigue
- headache
- poor appetite
- an unusual, streaked rash
- swollen glands, especially around the head, neck and arms
- gastritis
- lower abdominal pain

- sore soles
- tender subcutaneous nodules along the extremities
- lymph nodes may be enlarged and the throat can be sore

Signs and Symptoms of Ehrlichia

- sudden high fever
- fatigue
- muscle aches
- headache
- low white blood cell count
- low platelet count
- anemia
- elevated liver enzymes
- kidney failure
- respiratory insufficiency

Signs and Symptoms of Mycoplasma

- chronic fatigue
- joint pain
- intermittent fevers
- headaches
- coughing
- nausea
- gastrointestinal problems
- diarrhea
- visual disturbances
- memory loss
- sleep disturbances
- skin rashes
- joint stiffness
- depression
- irritability
- congestion
- night sweats
- loss of concentration

- muscle spasms
- nervousness
- anxiety
- chest pain
- breathing irregularities
- balance problems
- light sensitivity
- hair loss
- problems with urination
- congestive heart failure
- blood pressure abnormalities
- lymph node pain
- chemical sensitivities
- persistent coughing
- eye pain
- floaters in the eyes

Signs and Symptoms of Babesia

- high fever
- chills
- night sweats
- air hunger
- occasional cough
- persistent migraine-like headache
- sense of imbalance
- encephalopathy
- fatigue
- hemolysis

Signs and Symptoms of Candida

- sore, inflamed mouth and/or tongue
- burning tongue
- itchy ears
- itching of the skin
- outbreaks of eczema and/or psoriasis

- chronic sore throat
- heartburn
- chronic bladder disorders
- vaginitis or thrush
- vaginal discharge
- abdominal cramps
- PMS
- ovarian cysts
- prostate inflammation
- mental fogginess
- fatigue
- fibromyalgia-like symptoms
- cold hands and feet
- sinus disorders
- bronchial disorders and/or asthma
- flu-like syndrome
- extreme sensitivity to fumes and chemicals
- cravings for sugar or sweets
- cravings for alcohol, especially wine and beer
- chronic constipation
- alternating constipation and diarrhea
- spastic colon and/or irritable bowel syndrome

Lyme Disease Mimics

- acrodermatitis chronica atrophicans (ACA)
- Alzheimer's disease
- Bell's palsy
- Parkinson's disease
- irritable bowel syndrome
- lupus
- reflex sympathetic dystrophy
- scleroderma
- syphilis
- acute atrioventricular block
- arrhythmia

- attention deficit disorder
- attention deficit hyperactivity disorder
- Tourette's syndrome
- cranial polyneuritis
- chronic depression
- anxiety neurosis
- encephalopathy
- insomnia and other sleeping disorders
- myopia
- macular degeneration
- meningitis
- myocarditis
- cardiomyopathy
- neuritis
- chronic fatigue syndrome
- fibromyalgia
- tendinitis
- synovitis
- single joint arthritis
- rheumatoid arthritis
- Guillain-Barré Syndrome
- ALS
- polymyalgia rheumatic
- MS
- schizophrenia
- leaky gut syndrome

Bibliography

Aguero-Rosenfeld, M.E., et al. 2005. Diagnosis of lyme borreliosis. *Clin Microbiol Rev.* 18:484.

Asbrink, E., Hoymark, A., and B. Hederstedt. 1984. The spirochetal etiology of acrodermatitis chronica atrophicans Herxheimer. *Acta Derm Venereol.* 64:506-12.

Bale, J.F., Jr. and J.R. Murph. 1992. Congenital infections and the nervous system. *Pediatr Clin North Am* 39: 669-90.

Brown, J.S. Jr. 1994. Geographic correlation of schizophrenia to ticks and tick-borne encephalitis. *Schizophr Bull.* 20(4):755-75.

Brzostek, T. 2004. Human granulocytic ehrlichiosis co-incident with Lyme borreliosis in pregnant woman—a case study. *Przegl Epidemiol.* 58:289-94.

Burrascano, J.J., Jr. 2008. Advanced Topics in Lyme Disease. (Available as an Internet PDF, ilads.org)

Carlomagno, G., Luksa, V., Candussi, G., Rizzi, G.M. and G. Trevisan. 1988. Lyme Borrelia positive serology associated with spontaneous abortion in an endemic Italian area. *Acta Eur Fertil* 1988 Sep-Oct;19(5):279-81 Dept. of Obstetrics and Gynecology, University of Trieste School of Medicine.

Carroll, M.C. 2003. Lab 257: *The Disturbing Story of the Government's Secret Plum Island Germ Laboratory*. New York: Harper-Collins.

Chmielewski T., et al. 2003. Improvement in the laboratory recognition of lyme borreliosis with the combination of culture and PCR methods. *Mol Diagn.* 7:155-62.

Clark, K.L., Leydet, B., and S. Hartman. 2013. Lyme borreliosis in human patients in Florida and Georgia, USA. *Int J Med Sci.* 10:915-31.

Dandache, P. and R.B. Nadelman. 2008. Erythema migrans. *Infect Dis Clin North Am.* 22:235.

Dattwyler, R.J. and J.J. Halperin. 1987. Failure of tetracycline therapy in early Lyme disease. *Arthritis Rheum.* Apr;30(4):448-50.

Dupuis, M.J. 1988. Multiple neurologic manifestations of *Borrelia burgdorferi* infection. *Rev Neurol* (Paris) 144:765-75.

Embers, M.E., Barthold, S.W., Borda, J.T., Bowers, L., Doyle, L., and E. Hodzic. 2012. Persistence of Borrelia burgdorferi in Rhesus Macaques following Antibiotic Treatment of Disseminated Infection. *PLoS ONE.*
http://www.plosone.org/article/info%3Adoi%2F10.1371%2Fjournal.pone.0029914.

Fallon, B.A., Kochevar, J.M., Gaito, A, and J.A. Nields. 1998. The underdiagnosis of neuropsychiatric Lyme disease in children and adults. Ljdschr Geneeskd. 1993 Oct9;137(4):2098-100. *Psychiatr Clin North Am*. Supp;21(3):693-703, viii.

Gardner, T. 1995. *Lyme disease. Infectious diseases of the fetus and newborn infant.* (In) J. S. Remington and J. 0. Klein. Philadelphia, Saunders. Chap. 11: 447-528.

Goldenberg, R.L and C. Thompson. 2003. The infectious origins of stillbirth. *Am J Obstet Gynecol* 189: 861-73.

Grier, T.E. 2000. *Lyme Disease Survival Manual*. Duluth, MN.

Gustafson, J.M., Burgess, E.C., et al. 1993. Intrauterine transmission of *Borrelia burgdorferi* in dogs. *Am J Vet Res* 54(6): 882-90. (dog study)

Hercogova, J. and D. Vanousova. 2008. Syphilis and borreliosis during pregnancy. *Dermatol Ther*. 2008 May-Jun;21:205-9.

Klempner, M., et al. 2001. Two controlled trials of antibiotic treatment in patients with persistent symptoms and a history of Lyme disease. *The New England Journal of Medicine*. 345:85-92.

MacDonald, A.B. 1989. Gestational Lyme borreliosis. Implications for the fetus. *Rheum Dis Clin North Am* IS:657-77.

MacDonald, A.B. 1986. Human fetal borreliosis, toxemia of pregnancy, and fetal death. *Zentralbl Bakteriol Mikrobiol Hyg* [A] 263:189-200.

MacDonald, A.B., et al. 1987. Stillbirth following maternal Lyme disease. *NYState J Med* 87: 615-6.

Mattman, L.H. 2001. *Cell Wall Deficient Forms*. Boca Raton, FL: CRC Press.

McCarrison, R.M. 1927. *Studies in Deficiency Disease*. London: Oxford Univ. Press.

Middelveen, M.J., et al. 2014. Granulomatous hepatitis associated with chronic *Borrelia burgdorder* infection: a case report. *Research Open Access*. 1:875.

Middelveen, M.J., et al. 2014. *Journal of Investigative Medicine*. 62:280.

Moorcroft, T. *Internet publications*, www.originsofhealth.com.

Murray, R.I., Morawetz, R., Kepes, J., el Gammal, T. and M. LeDoux. 1992. Lyme neuroborreliosis manifesting as an intracranial mass lesion. *Neurosurgery*. 30:769-73.

Nicolson, G.L., Nicolson, N.L. and J. Haier, 2008. Chronic Fatigue Syndrome Patients Subsequently Diagnosed with Lyme Disease Borrelia burgdorferi: Evidence for Mycoplasma species Co-Infections. *Journal of Chronic Fatigue Syndrome*. 14: 5-17.

Ratnasamy N.I., Everett, E.D., Rolane, W.E., McDonald, G. and C.W. Caldwell. 1996 Central nervous system manifestations of human ehrlichiosis. *Clin Infect Dis*. Aug;23(2):314-9.

Romero, Luis M.D., PhD. 2003. Neurotoxins Focus. *Allergy Research Group Newsletter* pg.10 Oct.

Schlesinger, P.A. and P.H. Duray, et al. 1985. Maternal-fetal transmission of the Lyme disease spirochete, Borrelia burgdorferi. *Ann Intern Med* 103: 67-8.

Sherr, V.T. 2004. Human babesiosis–an unrecorded reality. Absence of formal registry undermines its detection, diagnosis and treatment, suggesting need for immediate mandatory reporting. *Med Hypotheses*. 63(4):609-15

Stricker, R.B. and L. Johnson. 2013. Persisent infection in chronic Lyme disease: does form matter? *Int. Lyme and Assoc. Disease Soc.* http://www.hoajonline.colm/journals/pdf/2052-5958-1-2.pd

Weber, K., and Bratzke, H.J., et al. 1988. *Borrelia burgdorferi* in a newborn despite oral penicillin for Lyme borreliosis during pregnancy. *Pediatr Infect Dis* J 7:286-9.

Williams, C.L., Strobino, B.A. and A. Lee, et al. 1990. Lyme disease in childhood: Clinical and epidemiologic features of ninety cases. *Pediatr. Infect*. Dis., 9:10–14.

Williams, C.L. and B.A. Strobino. 1990. Lyme disease and pregnancy–A review of the literature. *Contemporary Ob/Gyn*, 35:48–64.

Wormser, G.P., Dattwyler, R.J., Shapiro, E.D., Halperin, J.J., Steere, A.C., and M.S. Klempner, et al. 2006. The clinical assessment, treatment, and prevention of lyme disease, human granulocytic anaplasmosis, and babesiosis: clinical practice guidelines by the Infectious Diseases Society of America. *Clin Infect Dis*. 43:1089

Van den Bergen, H.A., Smith, J.P., and A. van der Zwan. 1993. Lyme psychosis. *Ned Tijdschr Geneeskd*. Oct9;137(41):2098-100.

Index

A

ADHD, 244-245
Adrenal glands, 164, 165, 237
Alcohol, 62, 90, 116, 131, 142, 150, 186, 187, 215, 263
ALS, 33, 34, 89, 99, 103, 113, 115, 116, 118, 123-125, 156, 175, 264
Alzheimer's disease, 100, 103, 115, 118, 123, 125, 263
American Journal of Tropical Medicine and Hygiene, 77
American Lyme Disease Foundation, 38
Anaplasma, 43, 164, 167
Andrews, Barbara, J., 50
Angina, 84
Antibiotics, 16, 17, 19, 20, 24-28, 30, 35, 42, 58-62, 69-72, 74-76, 78, 81, 89, 93, 112, 117, 118, 123, 125, 129, 130, 133, 134, 147, 152, 171, 172, 186, 246, 247, 253
Anxiety, 72, 98, 100, 120, 123, 124, 125, 154, 171, 175, 195, 257, 262, 264
Apoptosis, 57, 113, 114
Arthritis, 29, 31, 54, 98, 144, 183
  juvenile, 38, 245, 257
  rheumatoid, 15, 40, 54, 99, 101, 146, 170, 264
  single joint, 55, 56, 99, 264
Arthritis and Rheumatism, 19
Arthritis and Rheumatology, 156

B

Babesia, 27, 43, 128, 164, 172, 173, 250, 251, 262
Bartonella, 16, 31, 86, 128, 164, 169, 172, 244, 250, 251, 260
B complex, 27, 81, 83, 95, 119, 127, 136, 139-143, 193, 195-198
Bell's palsy, 33, 34, 98, 100, 121, 245, 258, 263
Biofilm, 75, 76
Bioterrorism, 39, 103
Biowarfare research, 103, 106
Bioweapons, 47, 53, 104, 109
Black seed oil, 81, 119, 126, 202
Bloodstream, 9, 42, 51, 76, 152, 163, 195
Bone activating complex, 128, 138-140, 142, 200, 255
Borrelia burgdorferi, 14, 30, 43, 49, 51, 69, 78, 114, 176
Bullseye rash, 8, 9, 160, 245, 257
Burbot oil, 119, 200, 201

C

Candida albicans, 59, 60-63, 65
  symptoms of, 61, 62
  protocol for, 63-64
Cardiac Lyme, 8, 84, **153-155** see also Lyme
Cardiomyopathy, 34, 100,
Carrot juice, 188
Carvacrol, 22
Cat's claw, 81, 112, 117, 119, 126, 127, 136, 138, 139, 141, 146-148
Cell phones, 177, 178
Cell Wall Deficient Forms: Stealth Pathogens, 114
Cell wall deficient organisms, 71
CFS (chronic fatigue syndrome), 115
Chaga, 79, 81, 93, 119, 120, 127, 128, 131, 136, 139-143, 155, 158, 159, 202, 247
Chronic fatigue syndrome, 34, 52, 99, 105, 106, 115, 116, 175, 245, 264
Cholesterol, 119, 176, 201, 202
Cinnamon oil, 25, 59
Co-infections, 14-16, 24, 27, 29, 80, 91, 128, 134, 146, 167, 172, 188
Cumin oil, 24, 63, 65, 129, 135, 162

D-E

Deer tick, 8, 13, 15, 33, 42, 94, 152
Depression, 34, 72, 98, 100, 120, 195, 258, 261, 264

Diabetes, 29

Diarrhea, 62, 76, 98, 129, 130, 175, 259, 261, 263
Dietary poisons, 180-181
Ecologic 500, 26, 63, 87, 136-139, 141
Ehrlichia, 16, 31, 43, 128, 164, 167, 168, 172, 261
Ehrlichiosis, 167
Encephalitis, 16, 32, 118, 151-153, 169, 171
Exercise, 129, 178-180, 252
Exhaustion, 31, 68, 105, 164, 174

F

Factor X, 193 see also Burbot oil; Omega-ADK; Freshwater cod
Fatigue, 19, 31, 34, 52, 61, 86, 87, 99, 101, 104-106, 115, 116, 130, 174-176, 195, 245, 260-264
Fibromyalgia, 34, 52, 61, 99, 116, 156, 245, 263, 264
Freshwater cod, 81, 139, 140, 142, 201, 255
Fukushima, 191, 197, 209
Fungus, 59, 60, 64, 186

G

Genital Lyme, **160** see also Lyme
Georgetown University, 23, 64, 78
Gluten, 181-185
GMOs, 22, 23, 150, 189, 191, 196, 200
Greens, 136, 138-146, 197, 199, 200
Grier, T.M., 29
Guillain-Barré, 33, 85, 99, 264
Gulf War syndrome, 175

H

Headache, 32, 70, 98, 111, 120, 125, 130, 168, 174, 176, 258-262
Hepatitis, 162, 163
Herbal Tick-X, 68, 95, 96, 252, 255
Herxheimer response, 129, 130, 150
Hormonal dysregulation, 164
Howenstine, Jones, 103, 105

I

Immune system, 16, 27, 30, 34, 42, 46, 58, 60, 63, 71, 73, 75, 82, 99, 102, 121, 133, 173, 179, 180, 182, 184, 187, 189, 195, 198, 249, 252
Insomnia, 100, 112, 120, 128, 171, 257, 264
Ioxides scapularis, 8 see also Deer tick

J

Joint
- disease, 8, 40, 45, 54, 55, 56, 160
- pain, 174, 176, 245, 259, 261
- stiffness, 98, 101, 257, 259, 261
- swelling, 56, 130, 183, 245

Jones, C. Ray, M.D., 245-247
Journal of Degenerative Diseases, 51
Journal of Neuroinflammation, 113

K-L

Kuppfer cells, 163
Lab 257: The Disturbing story of the Government's Secret Plum Island Germ Laboratory, 106
Lippia gravolens, 20
Lone star tick, 76, 77, 107, 168, 176
Lupus, 29, 100, 263
Lyme
- cardiac, 8, 84, 142, 153, 154
- muscular, 155, 158
- neurological, 111, 128
- genital, 160
- hepatitis, 162, 163

Lyme Disease Survival Manual, 29

M

MacDonald, Alan, M.D., 124
Mattman, Lida, 114-116, 159
McCarrison, Robert, 143, 144
MCHC, 138-140

Mechanisms of Microbial Disease, 54
Mental confusion, 120
Misdiagnosis, 34
Moorcroft, T., 13, 164, 244
Mosquitoes, 41, 48, 52, 250, 251
Multiple sclerosis (MS), 33, 34, 89, 99, 103, 113, 104, 115, 118, 120, 123, 125, 245, 175, 264
Muscular Lyme, 155-160 *see also* Lyme
Mycoplasma, 16, 31, 52, 86, 115, 120, 128, 164, 172, 174-176, 202, 250, 251, 261
Mycoplasma fermentans, 16, 51, 52, 250
Mycotoxins, 65, 74

N

Nervous system, 9, 13, 29, 32-34, 57, 70, 86, 89, 91, 101, 102, 111, 113, 116, 118, 121, 122, 125, 127, 147, 153, 157, 171, 174, 178, 196, 247
Neuroborreliosis, 70, 86, 99, 102, 111, 112, 113, 117, 121-123, 142, 176, 187
Neurological Lyme, **111-128** see also Lyme
Neuropathy, 19, 34, 118
Neurosurgery, 118
Neurotoxins, 77, 124
Noguchi, 99
North Carolina Health News, 170

O

Omega-ADK, 139, 140, 142, 201 see also Burbot oil
Operation Paperclip, 50 see also Plum Island
Origanum vulgare, 21, 65

P

Pandemic, 7, 11, 13, 14, 37, 39, 47, 104, 106, 107, 108, 246
Paralysis, 19, 32-34, 85, 100, 120, 122-124, 149, 155, 156, 175, 176, 258
Parasites, 15, 31, 43, 134, 175
Parkinson's disease, 100, 103, 104, 115, 118, 123, 125, 263
Pericarditis, 34
Peyer's Patches, 73-75, 182
Plum Island, 47-56, 94, 104, 106-110, 247, 254
Polymyositis, 34
Powasson encephalitis, 151, 164
Premarin, 115
Probiotics, 25-27, 59
Protocol,
  candida yeast, 63, 64
  nervous system Lyme infection, 125-128
Pseudomonas auregenosa, 22

R

Ramesh, G., 113, 114
Red sour grape powder, 84, 119, 136, 142, 214, 223
Relapses, 34, 102
Rhus coriaria, 24, 63, 65, 78, 81, 82, 130, 138-141, 247, 255
Rickettsia, 15, 28, 43, 52, 152
Rockefeller Institute, 104
Rocky Mountain Spotted Fever, 52, 93
Rodents, 31, 41, 43, 53, 68, 163, 169, 170

S

Savage, Harry, M.D., 76, 77
Secretory IgA, 182, 194
Seizures, 120, 170, 171, 260
Sigurdson, Bjorn, Dr., 104
Snydman, D.R., 54
Spinal cord, 9, 16, 32, 33, 79, 89, 102, 111, 112, 113, 117, 121, 122, 151, 156, 157, 175, 178, 247
Spice oils, 17, 24, 59, 60, 62, 64, 65, 79, 95, 101, 117, 118, 122, 129, 131, 156, 158, 162, 250, 252, 253, 244, 246, 247

Sponaugle Wellness Institute, 72, 73
STARI, 176
Steroids, 34, 164
Stiffness of neck, 98, 112, 120, 258
Stiffness of spine, 70, 98, 112

Stress, 16, 46, 60, 65, 79, 89, 102, 123, 125, 129, 157, 164, 176, 177, 179
Studies in Deficiency Disease, 143
Swelling, 31, 55, 56, 84, 87, 88, 90, 98, 101, 102, 130, 153, 155, 183, 195, 245, 257-259
Syphilis, 31, 34, 55, 99, 100, 102, 120, 160, 161, 243, 263

T

Teasel root, 81, 90, 127, 136-140, 142, 148-150, 255
The Body Shape Diet, 165
Thymus capitatus, 20, 21
Tick removal, 84, 131
TMJ, 32, 101, 257
Traub, Erich, 50, 52, 107, 108 see also Plum Island

V

Vitamin A, 81, 187-189, 241
Vitamin C, 82, 136, 138-143, 193, 197-200
Vitamin D, 82, 193, 198, 200
Vitamin K, 27, 189, 193, 200, 201

W-Z

West Nile virus, 39, 48, 106
Whitaker, Jo Anne, 100
Wild greens, 138-141, 143-146,
Wood ticks, 33, 94
Yeast, 57, 59-64, 69, 72-75, 95, 127, 186, 196